Can I Exercise Sitting Down?

I0414627

Can I Exercise Sitting Down?

Renee Wiggins

iUniverse, Inc.

New York Lincoln Shanghai

Can I Exercise Sitting Down?

iUniverse books may be ordered through booksellers or by contacting:

iUniverse
2021 Pine Lake Road, Suite 100
Lincoln, NE 68512
www.iuniverse.com
1-800-Authors (1-800-288-4677)

Thanks for giving me permission: ©STOTT PILATES®, a subsidiary of Merrithew Corporation(Day 26) MyPyramid.gov USDA Center for Nutrition Policy and Promotion(pgs. 86–89) ClipArt from © MicroSoft Fitness Wholesale for use of the Dyna-Band® in the picture.

ISBN-13: 978-0-595-38647-5 (pbk)
ISBN-13: 978-0-595-83028-2 (ebk)
ISBN-10: 0-595-38647-4 (pbk)
ISBN-10: 0-595-83028-5 (ebk)

Printed in the United States of America

Have you ever said to yourself, "I wish I could exercise without my knees hurting," or "I'm too heavy to do cardio"? Have you ever wondered, "Can I get a good workout sitting down?"

Yes! You can burn calories and tone muscles while sitting. You can exercise on a train, plane, bus, or at your desk; you will never miss a workout again.

Over the past few years, many of my personal training clients have asked me the same question, "Can I exercise sitting down?"

At first, I didn't believe what I was hearing. I thought everyone loved the sweaty, breathtaking high of exercising. I was wrong. After a hard day at the office, my clients felt too stressed to work out. I found that hardcore exercise added to a stressful day leads to cranky people.

In response to my clients' needs, I began to approach their exercise programs differently. I included light- and heavy-day workouts, and incorporated yoga, stretching or Pilates, and ten-minute massages.

My clients were and are still pleased with the results they have been getting.

I wrote this book for those just beginning an exercise program and to motivate those who need a jumpstart on their exercise routine.

Here, you will find traditional physical exercises as well as some thought-provoking mental exercises to promote balance between physical, mental, and spiritual health.

Before you turn the page, get permission from your doctor to start this, or any, exercise program. My book offers guidelines only. It should not be taken as the sole solution.

Are you ready to get started? Let's go!

Can I Exercise Sitting Down?
I dedicate to my wonderful family, friends, and clients,
who inspired me to write this book.
Thanks,
Renee

CONTENTS

ACKNOWLEDGMENTS

Thanks, Lauren G., Kelly G., Janice M., Sandra K., and Dehlia J., for posing as models in my book. *Say "Cheese!"*

Thanks, Kathy D., for suggesting that I change the book to a thirty-day exercise plan.

Thanks, Pat, for locking me in a hotel room to write.

Thanks, Mom, for pushing me to continue with my book when I couldn't think any more. Also, thanks for giving me the stocking to continue with my leg exercises when I forgot my Dyna-Band®.

Thanks, Sis, for teaching me how to use the camera and computer. Without your help, I would still be struggling. Thanks for being there.

Thanks, Carole Brown, for your inspiration and for reviewing my techniques.

Thanks to all of my friends and colleagues for your inspiration.

Thanks, Jodi Stolove, owner of Chair Dancing® International Inc., for reviewing the book and providing suggestions to make it more user friendly.

And a special thanks to Lakita Crider, a friend who lent her support, drive, and creativity to helping me complete this project.

Short Story One

As I travel throughout the Washington DC area, the driver on the X8 route complains about his weight every time I see him. He reminds me that he is still waiting for my help in assembling his exercise equipment, which is still in the box, unopened. He claims that I'm responsible for his twenty-pound weight gain (I only train women). He says that the unopened box of equipment reminds him of how much weight he has gained and how he wishes to be thin.

Want to share your story?
Visit Results By Renee at www.resultsbyrenee.com

Out of the Box

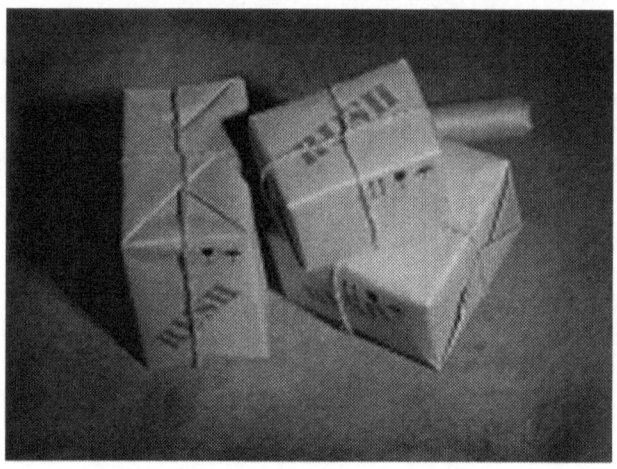

Remember when you had your new equipment shipped in a hurry—FedEx-ed or Priority Mailed—because you wanted to start exercising right away?

You couldn't wait. Some of you even stayed home to receive the package, while others left work early to see whether it had been delivered.

Is that equipment now hidden around the house, in a closet or in the garage?

Take it out of the closet!
Take it out of the box!
Unwrap it, unfold it, assemble it, and set it up!

If you are using a treadmill as a storage rack for magazines, newspapers, or clothes, remove them. If you are using the treadmill as a plant stand, remove the plants, too. Dust the treadmill off.

Now, use it!

Equipment

Dumbbell Weights:

Choose a weight that allows you to do ten bicep curls without getting tired in the first set.

Gradually increase the weight by five-pound increments when you feel the exercise has become too easy.

Dyna-Band® Exercise Bands:

Are available in various colors to represent different strengths/resistances.

Pink: Least Resistance
Green: Medium Resistance
Purple: Greatest Resistance

Dyna-Band®   are   available   for   purchase   at <u>*www.resultsbyrenee.com*</u>

Dyna-Band® and the Associated Colors are trademarks of The Hygenic Corporation. Unauthorized use is strictly prohibited.

Mat:

Exercise mats add comfort and support to your exercise.

Bottle of Water:

Water prevents dehydration from fluid lost during exercise.

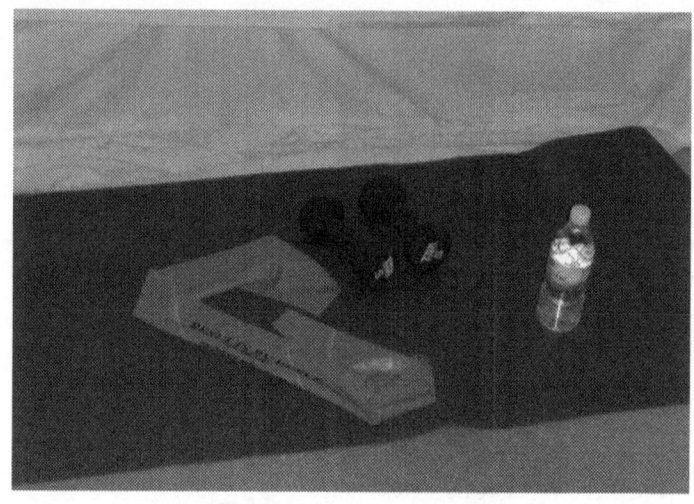

Dumbells, water bottle, and Dyna-Band®

Excuses, Excuses, Excuses

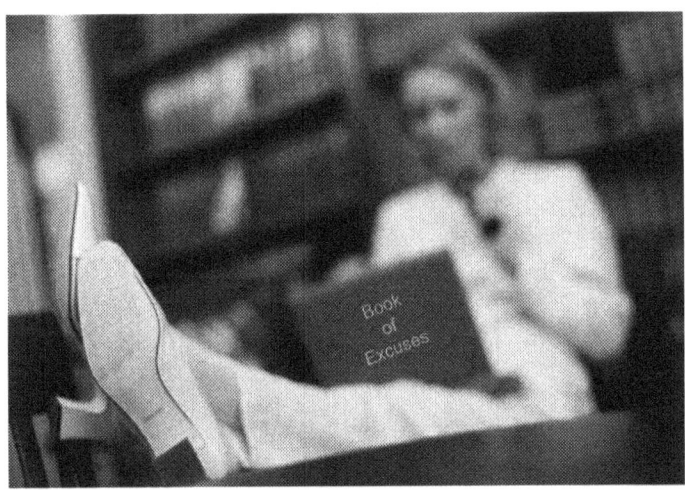

Drop These Excuses	Pick Up These Behaviors
"I don't want to sweat."	Take a Pilates or yoga class. Take a walk.
"I don't want to have sweaty hair."	Take the 10,000-Step Challenge. Wear a pedometer and record your number of steps at the end of the day.
	10,000 steps = 5 miles
"I don't have the time."	Exercise for ten minutes before work or after work. You don't have to exercise for a full hour.
"I don't want to shower…*again.*"	Exercise for ten minutes before showering for work or going to bed.

"I don't have the money for a gym membership or personal trainer."	Dust off the Hula Hoop®. Jump rope with the kids. Play kickball. Buy a mat (price range $5 to $10) and do floor exercises.
"I don't have time because I have to go to Bible class (or choir rehearsal, book club, girls' night out)."	Exercise before Bible class. You will feel fed in mind and spirit. Host a two-hour book club meeting. Dedicate the first hour (or thirty minutes) to exercising. You will be surprised at how clear your mind will become.
"I was at my mother's house (or traveling) and forgot my Dyna-Band®."	This happened to me. My mom told me, "I have some old stockings you can use." Guess what? *It worked.*

Write two excuses for why you can't (or don't want to) exercise. Then write two creative solutions for how you can exercise.

_____   _____

_____   _____

Guidelines for Dyna-Band® and Weights

Always remember to include safety as part of your fitness program. Whether you use the Dyna-Band® or weights, exercise caution.

The Dyna-Band® can be used almost anywhere. You can fold it and carry it with you easily on a plane, train, or bus, which is not possible with most weights. The Dyna-Band® promotes muscular strength and endurance, and increases range of motion.

Definitions

Muscular Strength: The ability to perform one repetition with maximum resistance.

Muscular Endurance: The ability to perform an exercise repetitively without getting tired.

Sets: The number of repetitions per muscle per exercise.

Repetitions or reps: The number of times you do one activity per muscle group.

Safety Precautions

- Do not let children play with the Dyna-Band® or weights.

- If you have high blood pressure (hypertension) be aware that resistance training can raise your blood pressure. Consult with your doctor before starting your resistance program.

- When placing the Dyna-Band® under your foot, always make sure you have at least two inches of the band under the foot. Press firmly to prevent the band from slipping and hitting you.

- To reduce the potential for injury, I recommend that you consult with a personal trainer on proper form whenever possible.
- If you suffer from carpal tunnel syndrome, consult with your doctor before performing the following exercises.

Workout Tips

- Perform one to three sets of eight to ten repetitions each. Rest for thirty seconds between each set.
- Sit with your back straight, shoulders in alignment (not rounded), and abdominal muscles contracted.
- To prevent injuries, always warm up before using the Dyna-Band® or weights.
- Stretch after your workout.
- Do not lock your joints.
- Breathe naturally.
- Perform each move slowly.
- Most importantly, maintain control of your Dyna-Band®.

Care of the Dyna-Band®

- Store in a dark area.
- To prevent breakage, sprinkle the band with talcum powder once a month.
- Untie the Dyna-Band® when not in use.

Dos and Don'ts for Weights

- Do not grip weights too hard; it will raise your blood pressure.
- Do not slam or hit weights together because you could hurt yourself.

- Do not let children use weights under the age of eight years, children over eight years can use weight but with proper supervision.

- Do not drop weights on the floor. Paint chips may splatter or the weights may hit your feet.

- Do consult with your doctor before starting a resistance program.

Got Ten Minutes?

What is your excuse not to exercise? No time? Do you have ten minutes? Grab a seat and a Dyna-Band® exercise band, and perform at least one of these exercises for ten minutes.

Exercise One: (Bicep Curl)

(Perform three sets of eight to ten repetitions. Rest between sets for thirty seconds.)

1. Place the Dyna-Band® exercise band under your right foot.
2. Hold the Dyna-Band® in your hands, palms up, at waist height.
3. Grasp Dyna-Band® with fingers closed.
4. Raise arms to shoulder height, keeping elbows at the waist, and exhale.

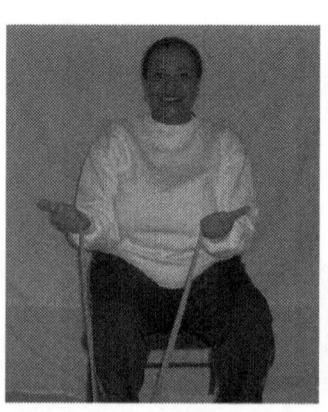
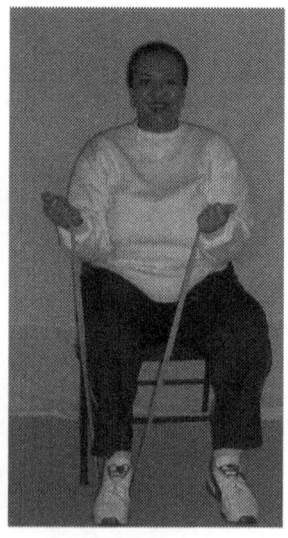

Exercise Two: Triceps Extension

(Perform three sets of eight to ten repetitions. Rest between sets for thirty seconds.)

1. Place the Dyna-Band® in your left hand; place hand on chest.
2. With your right hand, grasp the Dyna-Band®. Your right arm should be up and four inches away from your left arm.
3. Extend your right hand away from your left. Right arm should be perpendicular to the floor.
4. Keeping tension on the Dyna-Band®, return it to your left hand. Hands should not touch.
5. Extend right arm again, about eight inches away from your left hand.

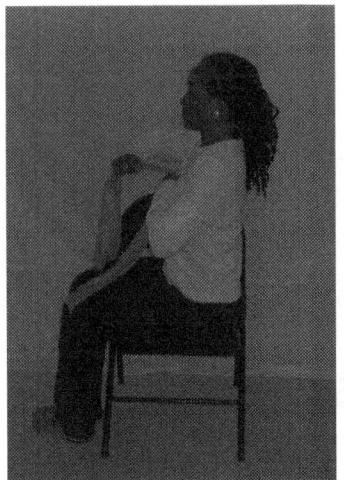
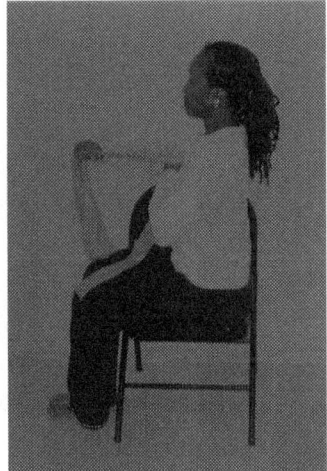

Exercise Three: Deltoid Extension

(Perform three sets of eight to ten repetitions. Rest between sets for thirty seconds.)

1. Place the Dyna-Band® band under your right foot. Make sure there are two inches of the band under your foot. Press firmly so the band will not move.

2. Grasp band with fingers pointed down.

3. Place your right hand and arm at your side with elbows straight and aligned at your waist.

4. Extend your right arm to the side and away from your body and exhale.

5. Slowly return to starting position.

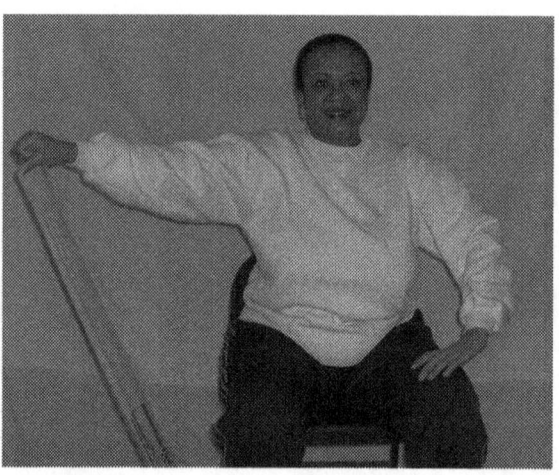

Perform at least one of the exercises above at your desk or in your favorite chair, and you will be amazed at how much you can do in just ten minutes.

Exercise Calendar

Suggestion: Make a copy of this calendar and post it where you can see it easily.

Instructions and illustrations for these exercises are included in the pages to follow.

SUNDAY	MONDAY	TUESDAY	WEDNESDAY	THURSDAY	FRIDAY	SATURDAY
Day 1 Walk, Treadmill, or Bike	Day 2 Stretching	Day 3 Biceps, Triceps	Day 4 Walk or Bike & Stretch	Day 5 Biceps, Triceps & Abs	Day 6 Stretch or Yoga	Day 7 Rest
Day 8 Biceps & Triceps	Day 9 Abs	Day 10 Walk	Day 11 Stretch or Yoga	Day 12 Meditate	Day 13 Biceps, Triceps, & Abs	Day 14 Walk
Day 15 Stretch	Day 16 Biceps, Triceps, & Abs	Day 17 Stretch or Yoga	Day 18 Inner Thighs	Day 19 Reflexology	Day 20 Meditate	Day 21 Inner and Outer Thighs
Day 22 Walk & Stretch	Day 23 Abs	Day 24 Biceps, Triceps, & Legs	Day 25 Rest Stretch	Day 26 Biceps, Triceps, & Abs	Day 27 Walk, Stretch, & Inner and Outer Thigh	Day 28 Rest
Day 29 Stretch or Yoga	Day 30 Biceps, Triceps, & Abs	Day 31 Now It's Your Turn				

Exercise Log

Suggestion: Make a copy of this log and use it to track how many sets of each exercise completed daily.

Day	Exercise Listing 1	Exercise Listing 2	Exercise Listing 3	Exercise Listing 4	Exercise Listing 5	Exercise Listing 6	Exercise Listing 7	Exercise Listing 8	Exercise Listing 9	Exercise Listing 10	Exercise Listing 11
01											
02											
03											
04											
05											
06											
07											
08											
09											
10											
11											
12											
13											
14											
15											
16											
17											
18											
19											
20											
21											
22											
23											
24											

	Exercise Listing 1	Exercise Listing 2	Exercise Listing 3	Exercise Listing 4	Exercise Listing 5	Exercise Listing 6	Exercise Listing 7	Exercise Listing 8	Exercise Listing 9	Exercise Listing 10	Exercise Listing 11
25											
26											
27											
28											
29											
30											
31											

Exercise Tips

- Consult a healthcare provider before starting any exercise program.
- Warm up before beginning any type of exercise.
- Always perform exercises in a slow and controlled manner.
- Avoid holding your breath while performing exercises.
- Keep your back straight while exercising.
- Stop if you feel tired or experience any discomfort or pain.

The Benefits of Exercise

- Builds self-esteem.
- Increases endurance and stability.
- Strengthens muscles, tendons, ligaments, and bones.
- Boosts morale.
- Enhances flexibility.
- Improves mental and physical well-being.
- Helps you sleep better and feel better.
- Reduces tension and anxiety.
- Reduces high blood pressure, high cholesterol, and high blood glucose levels.
- Increases bone density.
- Accelerates your metabolism.

Tips for Staying Motivated

- Exercise with a partner.
- Work out to music.
- Vary your workout so you don't get bored.
- Invite friends over for an exercise party. Play an exercise tape and work out together.
- Record your progress.
- Reward yourself with tickets to a show or a new book. Don't reward yourself with food.

Day 1: Getting Started

Begin with a commitment.

Consult with your doctor first. Once she or he has given you the green light, find an aerobic activity that interests you.

Walking is a good, inexpensive exercise. If you can't walk outdoors, walk indoors. Walk at the local mall in the early morning hours, or at the local school track. Why not walk in your hallway? Better yet, take the stairs instead of the elevator.

Start a walking program on your block or in your apartment complex. Offer incentives to those who walk more than 2,000 steps in the first day.

Today's Focus: Walk for thirty minutes or 10,000 steps per day (approximately 5 miles).

Today's Snack: An apple

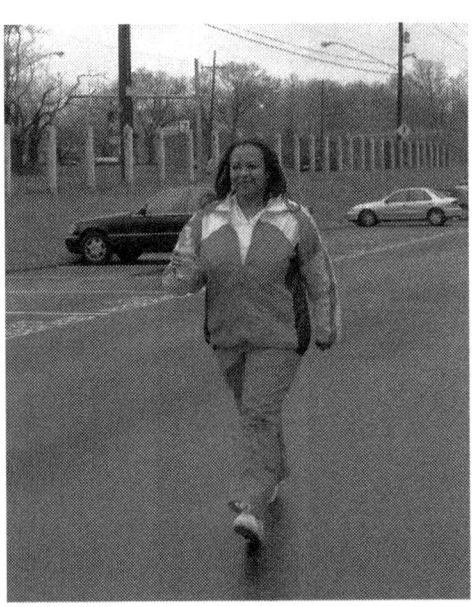

Day 2: Conversations with Self

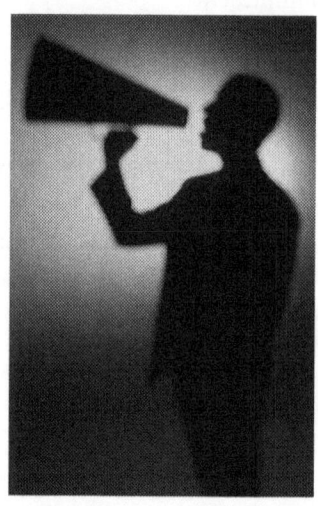

Did you know that constantly speaking or thinking words and phrases can cause you to believe them? Do you use words or phrases to hurt yourself?

Speak negatively, and you will live negatively.
"I am fat and can't do a thing."
"I can't eat small portions."

Speak positively, and you will think and live positively.
"I can exercise."
"I can lose weight."
"I can eat smaller portions."
"I can...I can...I can..."

Flexibility (stretching) exercises used to be neglected. Now everyone does them—stretching exercises, yoga, and Pilates. Stretching helps to increase your range of motion, allowing you to extend or bend farther. Stretching also reduces your risk of injuries.

Today's Focus: Stretch after a twenty-minute aerobic workout or after a hot bath. Stretching without first warming your muscles can cause injury. Warm muscles are more flexible.

Today's Snack: A small banana

How to: Stretch (lower back)

1. Sit with back against the chair.
2. Lean forward with feet flat on the floor and bend toward the floor.
3. Place your hands on the floor, if your hands cannot reach the floor hold onto your ankles, for support.

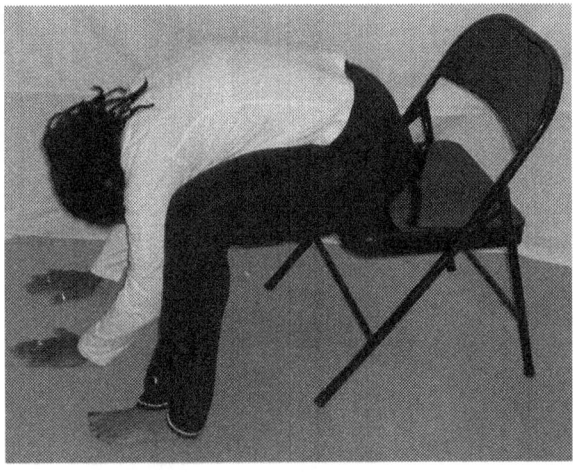

Day 3: Keep Exercising

You know the saying: "If at first you don't succeed, try, try again."

Keep on practicing. Don't give up.

Today's Focus: March in place for ten minutes or go for a walk. Stretch for two minutes.

Today's Snack: 1/2 cup of blueberries with 1/2 cup of low-fat yogurt.

How to: Bicep Curls

(Perform three sets of ten reps each. Rest thirty seconds between sets.)

1. Take a seat.

2. Hold weights at your sides with palms forward.

3. Inhale.

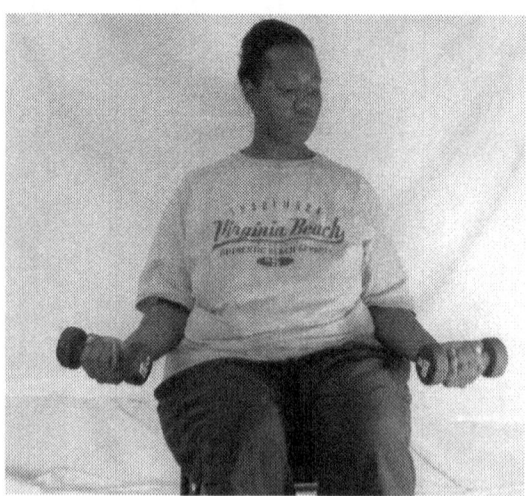

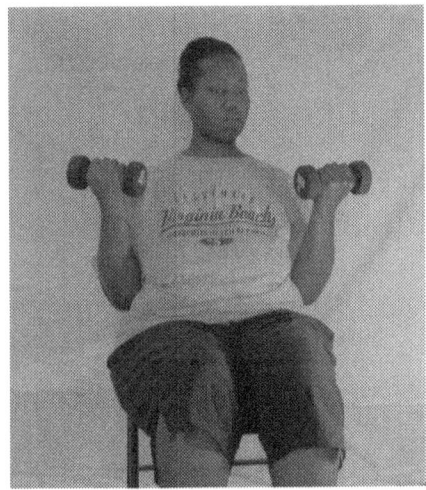

4. Raise weight and exhale.
5. Return to starting position and inhale.

How to: Triceps Kickback

(Perform three sets of ten reps each. Rest thirty seconds between sets.)

1. Place your left hand on a chair for balance.
2. Stand with left foot behind right foot.
3. Next your right hand to chest height and inhale.

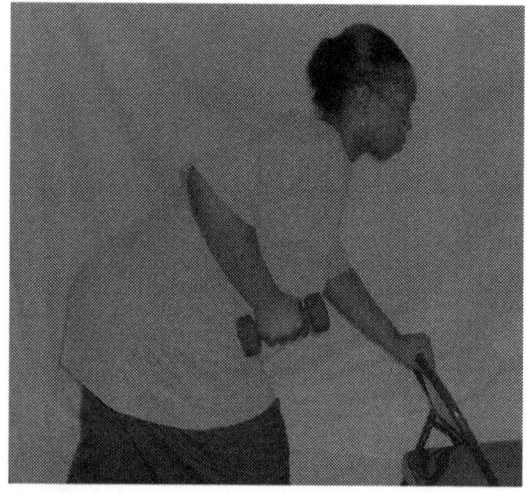

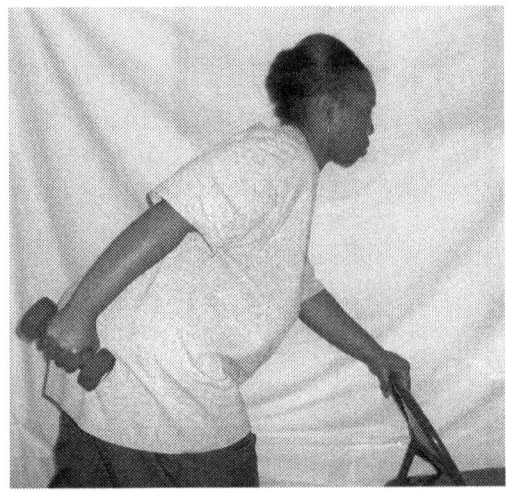

4. Extend your right hand behind you and exhale.
5. Keep your wrist straight.
6. Return to starting position and inhale.
7. Repeat on your left side.

Short Story Two

Mr. G., a fifty-six-year-old man weighing 309 pounds, came to me because he wanted to lose weight. I prescribed a 1,500-calorie diet, along with an exercise program.

I instructed Mr. G. in the use of weights to strengthen his biceps and triceps, and showed him exercises he could do while watching television (**Refer to Day 3**). By his tenth workout session, Mr. G. had lost four pounds simply by working out during commercial breaks. (His family thought he was doing too much because he even did bicep curls in the bathroom.)

Mr. G. was delighted with his results.

Want to share your story?
Visit Results By Renee at www.resultsbyrenee.com

Day 4: There Is Hope

I know you are tired of carrying your extra weight, wearing a smile to cover up your pain and frustration. *Today* there is hope you can change your body, change your dress size and you can change how you feel about yourself.

Today's Focus: Walk for twenty minutes.
Today's Snack: Fifteen grapes

How to: Stretch the Piriformis (hip rotator muscles)

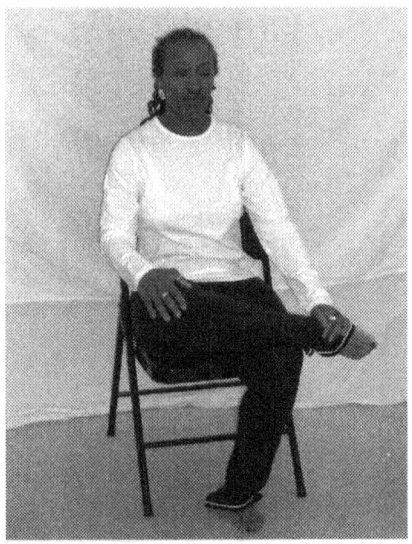

1. Sit in a chair with your back straight.

2. Cross your left leg over your right thigh.

3. Press your left hand down on your left knee to a point of discomfort.

4. Breathe naturally, and hold the stretch for ten to fifteen seconds.

Day 5: Are We There Yet?

Too many of us start an exercise or diet program on Monday expecting to reach our goals by Friday. Be patient. It takes time for your body to show changes.

You aren't there yet. Keep practicing.

Today's Exercises:

Biceps Curls: Three sets of ten reps each. Rest between sets. (**Refer to Day 3**)

Triceps Kickbacks: Three sets of ten reps each. Rest between sets. (**Refer to Day 3**)

Ab Sit-ups/Crunches: Three sets of twelve reps each. Rest between sets. (**See "How To," below**)

Today's Snack: 1/2 cup of light fruit cocktail with three graham crackers

How to: Abs (Sit-ups/Crunches)

1. Lie on the floor with knees bent.

2. Raise your arms behind your head and inhale.

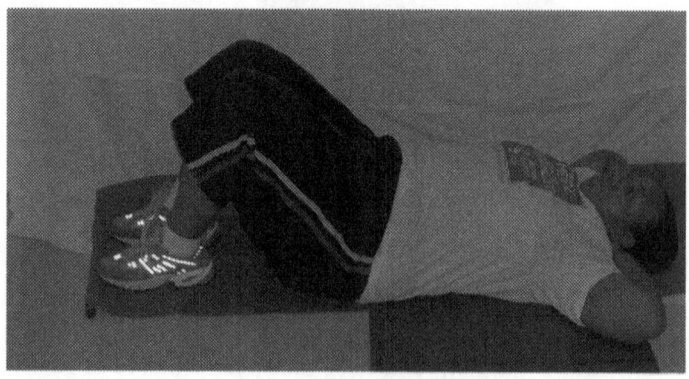

3. Raise your head and exhale.
4. Look straight at your knees.
5. Return to starting position and inhale.

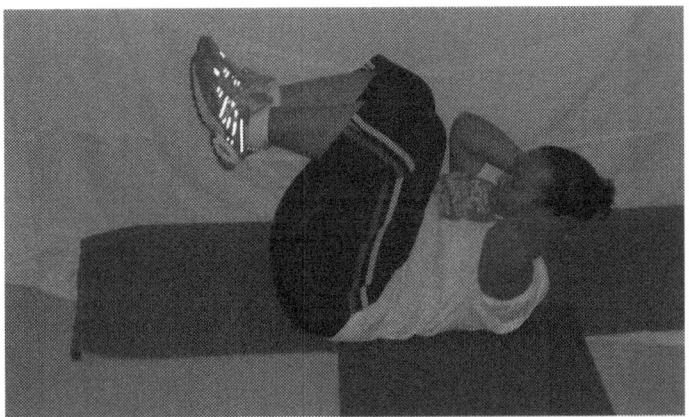

Day 6: Go with the Flow

Be in the moment. Don't let life's frustrations get you down. If nothing is going your way, maybe it shouldn't go your way. Go with the flow, and you will be surprised at how easy life can be.

Today's Focus: Warm up by walking for thirty minutes. Stretch.

Today's Snack: Ten baby carrots

How to: Stretch

This is a good stretch for your back.

1. Sitting with your knees bent at your hips.
2. Bend forward with arms reaching in front of you.
3. Breathe in and out your nose for ten to fifteen seconds.
4. Return to an upright position, sitting with knees bent.

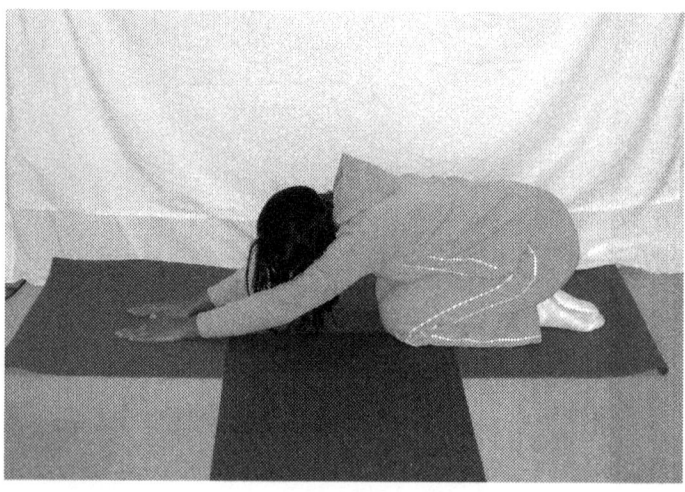

Day 7: Daring to Dream

Take time to dream. Visualize your dream. Determine to reach beyond the stars. Believe you can climb monumental mountains to achieve your dreams.

Rest.

Renew.

Rejuvenate.

Today's Focus: Stretch. Get a massage. Dare to dream.

Today's Snack: Indulge in 1/2 cup of low-fat pudding.

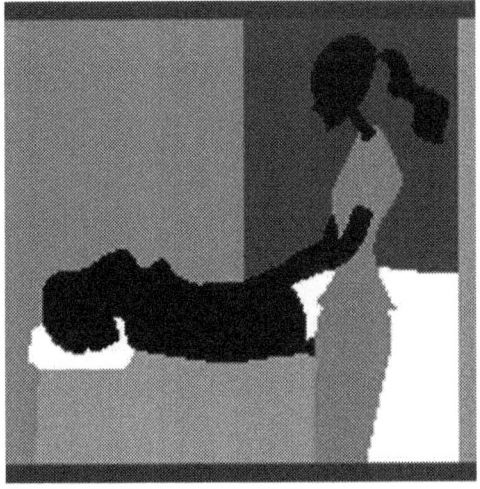

Day 8: Be SMART

<u>S</u>et <u>M</u>easurable <u>G</u>oals that can be <u>A</u>chievable in a <u>R</u>easonable <u>T</u>ime.

Don't set yourself up for failure. Be realistic. You can't lose twenty pounds in eight days or get a six-pack in less than a week. Start slowly and gradually increase your intensity. Remember to practice, practice some more, and keep on practicing.

Today's Focus:
Warm up for thirty minutes.
Biceps Curls: Three sets of twelve reps each. (**Refer to Day 3**)
Triceps Kickbacks: Three sets of twelve reps each. (**Refer to Day 3**)

Today's Snack: One cup of raw vegetables or fruit with 2 tbsp. of a low-fat dip

Day 9: Don't Quit

Quitters don't realize they are only five minutes away from their dreams.

Today's Focus: First, warm up by walking, running or aerobic dancing. Stretch. Reverse crunches and curl ups: three sets of ten reps each. If you cannot do ten repetitions, do three sets of eight reps until the exercise becomes easy. Gradually increase your repetitions.

Today's Snack: Two kiwi fruits and a 4-oz. glass of skim or soy milk

How to: Reverse crunches and curl ups

1. Lie on your back with knees bent, feet flat on the floor.
2. Place your hands behind your head while inhaling.

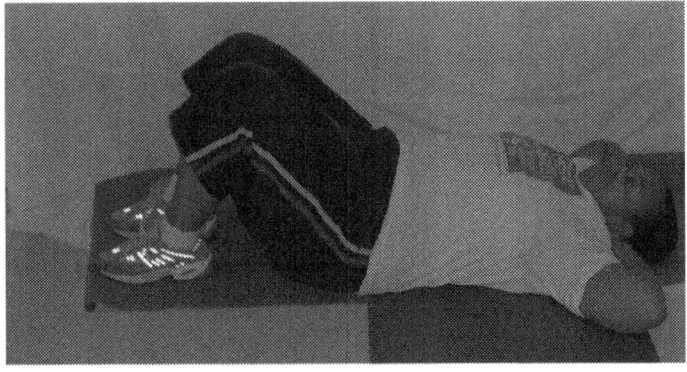

3. Bring knees and elbows together.
4. Exhale. (Do not squeeze your neck.)
5. Return to the starting position.

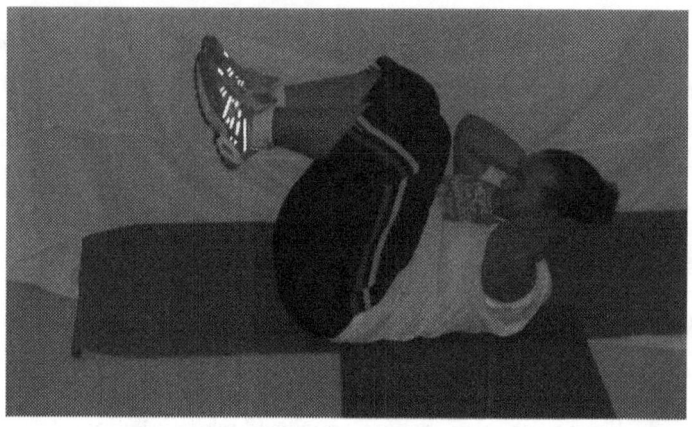

Short Story Three

I met B.B. ten years ago when she came to me for help with building her strength and maintaining her weight. She comes to me every other year to renew her exercise program while I review her form. She has gained strength and endurance and has successfully maintained her weight. Even during periods of stress, B.B. continues exercising but reduces her intensity.

Want to share your story?
Visit Results By Renee at www.resultsbyrenee.com

Day 10: "I Should Haves"

Don't waste your time on "I should have's."
"I should have gone to water aerobics three times a week."
"I should have bought that treadmill."
"I should have had a salad instead."

"I should have" is translated to
I—let
S—sorry
H—have a hold
O—on my
U—undivided attention
L—to lay down my life to be
D—dormant and uneventful.

Change. I should. I will.

Today's Focus: Walk for twenty-five minutes.
Today's Snack: 4 oz. of canned light pears

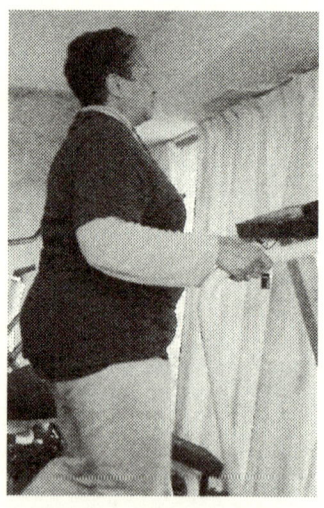

Day 11: Crossing the Bridge

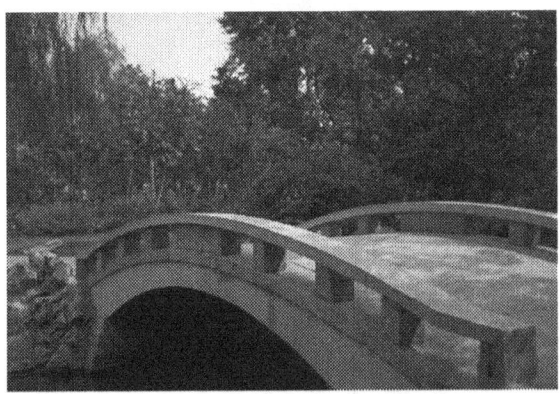

You find yourself crossing a bridge and wondering what is on the other side.
As you come close to the end, the bridge soon disappears.
And you wonder, why?

You start an exercise program and then *stop*.
You start a diet program, and soon you *stop*.
You buy an exercise tape and never remove the wrapper—you *stop*.
And you wonder, *Why?*

Is it because you don't want to reach the end?
Is it because the path is rocky and uneven?
Is it because everyone says you will not succeed?
And you wonder, *Why?*

No one says life, exercise, and dieting are without struggle or pain.
If the road were easy and painless, would you appreciate it more?

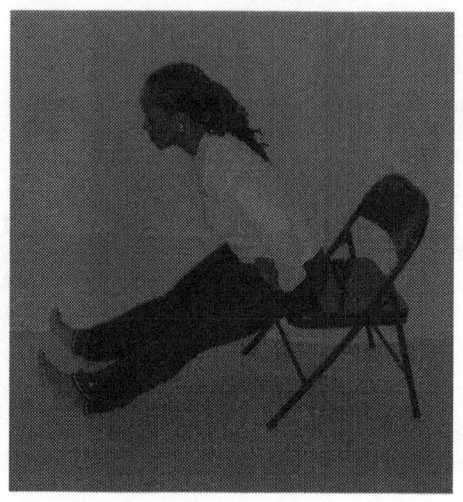

Today's Focus: Stretch (**Refer to Day 6**).
Today's Snack: 6-oz. fruit smoothie

How to: Calf and Hamstring Stretch

1. Sit on the edge of your chair.
2. Extend your feet forward with toes flexed.
3. Lean forward with your chest, keeping your head up.
4. Keep your back straight.
5. Breathe naturally.
6. Hold stretch for 10–15 seconds

Day 12: Stop Worrying

Don't let worrying become your god.

Focusing on your problems can lead to stress. Stress is an external force that can cause internal problems. It can be negative or positive, depending on how you look at it.

Negative stress can lead to sleepless nights, smoking, drinking, eating disorders, depression, ulcers, headaches, and more.

How do you handle stress?

Today's Focus: Change stress to a positive situation through prayer or meditation. First, stretch; then meditate. Light a candle and sit still for two minutes. Just stare at the candle. Don't let thoughts enter your mind. Just stare. Take time out for yourself *today*.

Today's Snack: An apple with 1 tbsp. of peanut butter

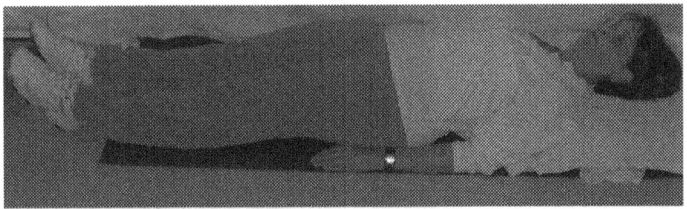

Day 13: Going Forward

Is exercise kicking your butt? Let it.

Every time exercise or something else kicks you in the butt, the only way to go is forward.

Today's Focus:

Bicep Curls: Three sets of twelve reps. Rest thirty seconds between sets. (**Refer to Day 3**)

Triceps Kickbacks: Three sets of twelve reps. Rest between sets. (**Refer to Day 3**)

Abs: Three sets of fifteen reps. Rest between sets. (**Refer to Day 5**)

Today's Snack: An orange

Day 14: Pop, Pop, *Pop*

We pop into our homes; pop something out of the freezer; pop it into the microwave; pop onto the sofa; start popping the remote control; and pretty soon, we are popping out of our clothes.

Today's Focus: Pop onto the treadmill or bike for forty-five minutes or more. Walk. Stretch after your workout. (**Refer to Days 6 and 11**)

Today's Snack: 4-oz glass of skim milk with two sugar-free cookies

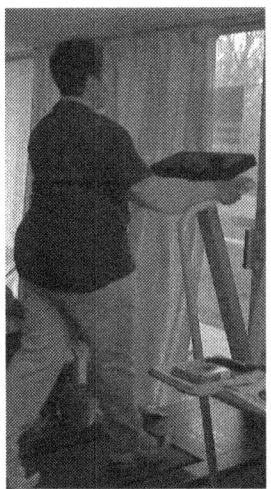

Day 15: The Halfway Mark

You are halfway there. Don't give up. Remember, exercise is a game of practicing until you get it right.

Today's Focus: Yoga

Today's Snack: An apple and ten nuts, such as almonds and peanuts

How to: "The Hero" meditation poses

1. Sit on your feet, keeping your knees together.
2. Keep your chest forward, with shoulders relaxed. And place hands on your thighs with palms facing upward with thumb and first finger touching. Do not lean back.
3. If this pose hurts your knees or feet, use a blanket between your heels and buttocks for support.
4. Breathe in and out your nose for two minutes.

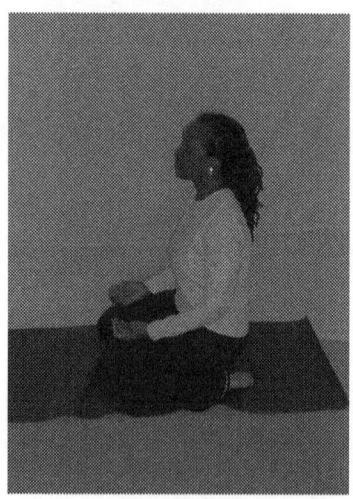

Day 16: Time Well Spent

It's only a few seconds between success and failure. How are you going to spend those seconds?

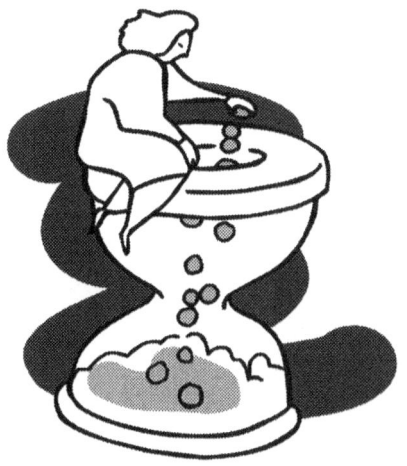

Today's Focus:
Biceps: Four sets of twelve reps. (**Refer to Day 3**)
Triceps: Four sets of twelve reps. (**Refer to Day 3**)
Abs: Three sets of twenty reps. (**Refer to Day 5**)

Today's Snack: One slice of whole-wheat bread with 1 tbsp. of peanut butter or one slice of cheese

How are you going to spend your seconds?

Seconds add up to minutes.
Minutes add up to hours.
Hours add up to days.
And days add up to months.

It takes ten seconds to monitor your blood glucose levels,
but you decided not to measure your blood glucose levels.
Those seconds have cost you a week in the hospital.

The doctor told you to take ten minutes to exercise,
but you decided to use those ten minutes to grab a Coke
and a bag of chips.
Now you are twenty pounds overweight.

How are you going to spend your seconds?

Day 17: Step Up to the Plate

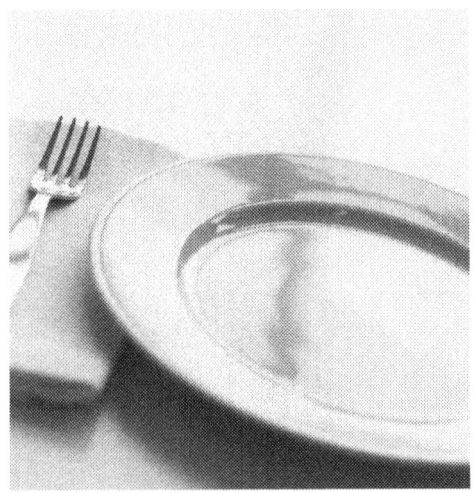

"Jack Sprat could eat no fat; his wife could eat no lean. And so, betwixt the both of them, they licked the platter clean."
—*Mother Goose Nursery Rhyme*

What is on your plate? Vegetables and starches should take up three-quarters of your plate. Protein and fat should take up the other quarter.

Today's Focus: Stretch the triceps muscles

1. Place your right hand over shoulder touching the middle of your back with palms down.

2. Place your left hand behind your back, touch the fingers on your right hand, if you can.

3. If your fingers don't quite touch, don't worry. With practice, they eventually will.

4. Hold the stretch for fifteen seconds.

Today's Snack: 1/2 cup of canned peaches

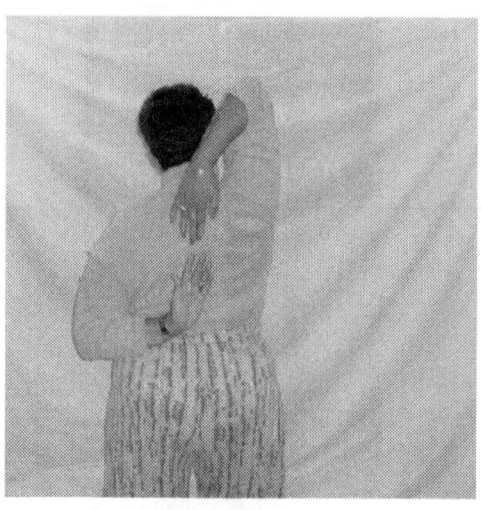

Day 18: Hey! You Still Can Exercise on the Couch

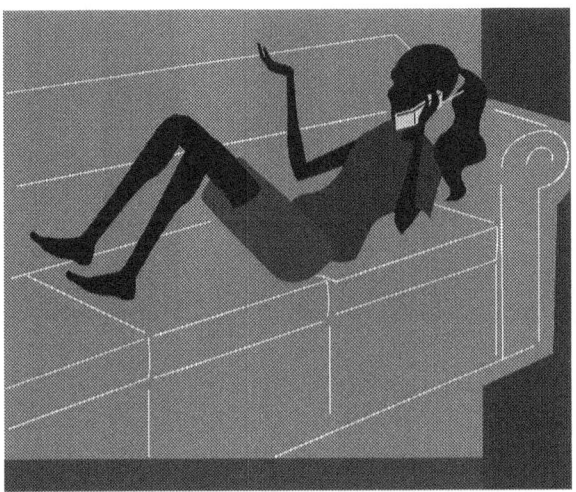

You have only fifteen more days to go!

Today's Focus: Warm up with a twenty-minute march in place. Stretch. (**Refer to Day 2**)

You can do leg-lifts while you are on the couch and keep talking, too.

Inner thigh exercises: (**Refer to Day 23**)

Today's Snack: 8-oz. glass of cocoa and two graham crackers

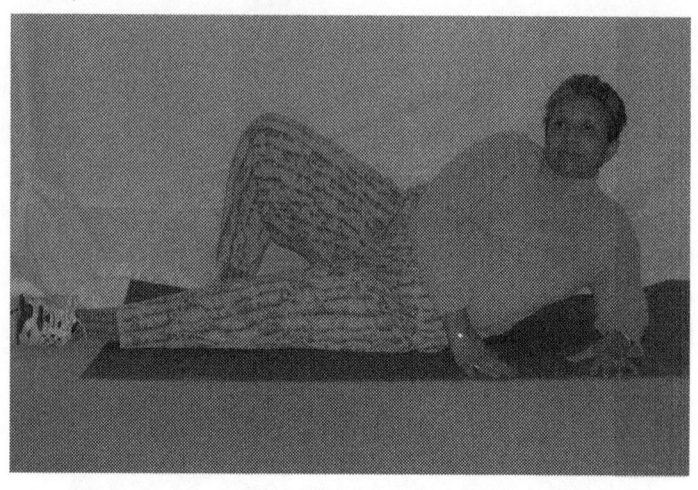

Day 19: Reflexology

Take a look at where you want to be. Visualize your goal, and determine how you are going to get there. Don't force it. It will only backfire in your face.

Whether it is inch by inch, step by step, pound by pound, or day by day, eventually you will get there.

Today's Focus: Treat yourself to a Reflexology session.

Reflexology is the art and science of applying pressure to the feet. Each pressure point has a therapeutic effect on a corresponding body part. The padding of your feet under your toes represents the chest and lung areas. The big toe represents your brain and the toes represent your sinus areas around your eyes and nose. Make an appointment to see a reflexologist. Have a relaxing foot massage.

Today's Snack: 6-oz. fruit yogurt and a nectarine

Day 20: Phew!

Yes, exercise is hard. Guess what? Life is also hard.

Think of your exercise program like giving birth. It takes time and needs constant care, and in the end a new *you* is born!

Exercise builds your morale, your self-esteem, and your character.

Rest and live your *best*!

Today's Focus: Take a break and meditate. Reflect on how far you have come, rather than how much more you have to achieve.

Today's Snack: 2 oz. of tuna packed in water, with five crackers

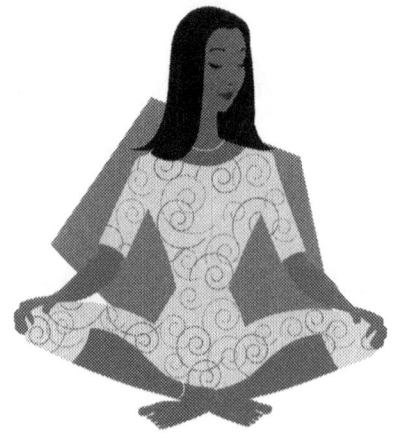

Day 21: Honor Yourself

"If you can't get from a size twenty-two to a size five, then size five is not for you."

Today's Focus:
Legs (Inner Thigh): Four sets of ten repetitions. Rest between sets for at least thirty seconds.

How to: Legs (Inner Thigh)

1. Start by lying on your left side.
2. Place hands on the floor in front of you.
3. Turn your front leg forward with your foot flexed.

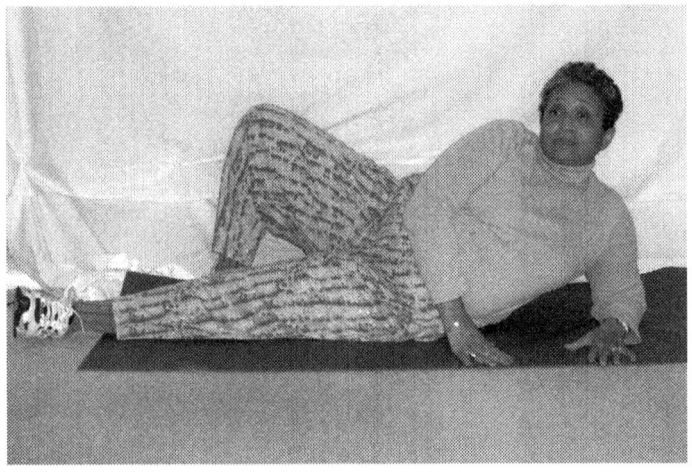

4. Raise your leg off the floor and exhale.

5. Return to the starting position and inhale.

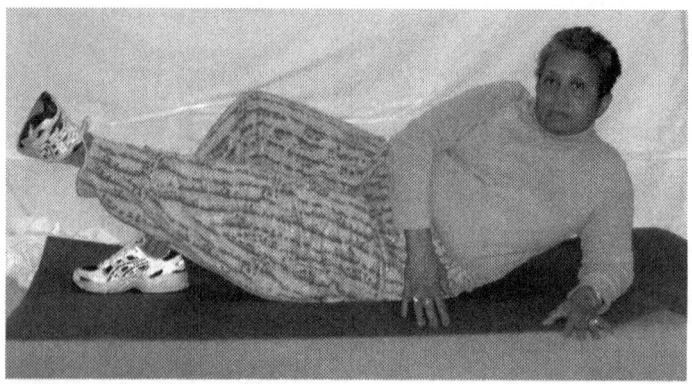

How to: Legs (Outer Thigh)

1. Lie on your side, head down.
2. You can either straighten the arm on the floor, or place that arm under your head.
3. Inhale. Raise leg off the floor. Exhale.
4. Return to starting position.

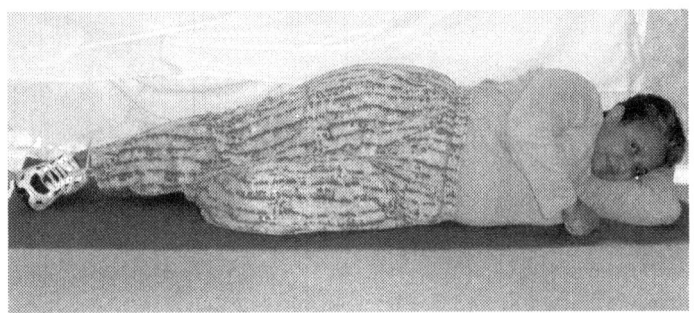

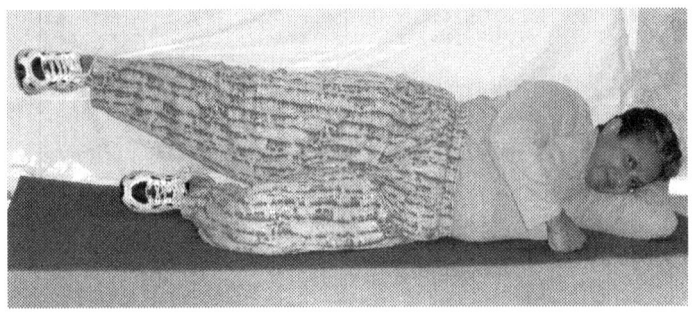

Today's Snack: One small apple and one slice of cheese

Day 22: I Saw *You*

I saw you the other day, running in the opposite direction.
I asked you to come and exercise with me.
You said, "I can't exercise because of my hair."

I saw you the other day, huffing and puffing, looking slightly
overweight.
I asked you to come along.
You said, "I can't exercise because I don't have the time."

I saw you the other day, coming out of the doctor's office
with a frown.
I asked you to come along.
You said, "I can't exercise because I don't like to sweat."

I saw you the other day, leaving Gwen's Crab Shack with two
boxes of crabs and another box of fried chicken wings and fries.
I asked you to come along.
You said, "I can't exercise because I have two DVDs to see."

I saw your sister the other day, looking slightly round, with a
frown, and huffing and puffing.
She told me they had to bury you the other day because you
died from diabetes complications.
I asked her to come along.
And she said, "_____"

What do you say?

Don't stop now. Keep on.

Today's Focus: Take a thirty-minute walk, and stretch.

Today's Snack: Three cups of popcorn

Day 23: Planning

To Fail to Plan is to Plan to Fail.

Make a *plan*. Plan to work. Work your plan. Plan to be successful.

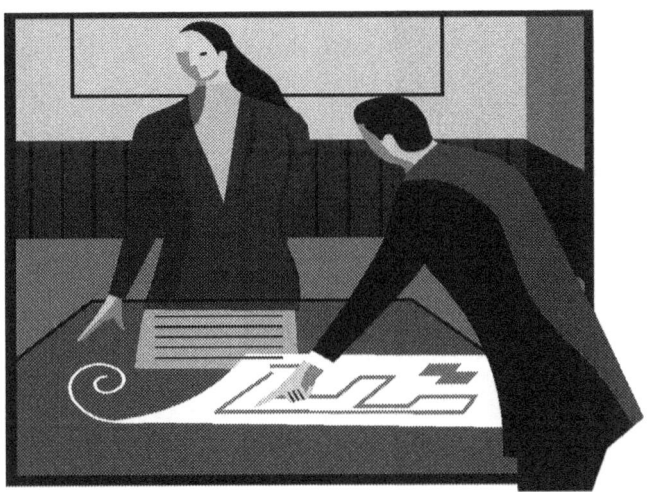

My Contract

My Plan:

(Fill in the blanks. *For example: I will drink just one 12-oz. soda per week.*)

I will lose___ pound(s) per week.
I will eat ___ calories per day.
I will eat ___ fruits per day.
I will eat ___ vegetables per day.
I will dine out ___ times a week.
I will perform sit-ups ___ times a week, ___ sets of ___ reps.

_____   _____
(Your signature)   (Witness Signature)

Follow this plan for 30 days.

Today's Focus: Abs/Sit-Ups
Do three to four sets of ten to twelve repetitions. Rest between sets. Then switch legs.

1. Lying on your back, cross your left leg over your right thigh.

2. Place your right hand under your head.

3. Extend your left arm to the left side of your body.

4. Inhale.

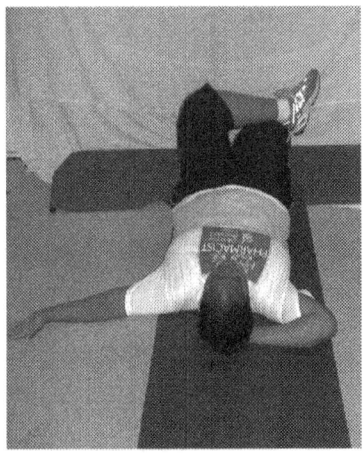

5. Raise your right arm to your left knee, while keeping your left arm on the floor. (Your elbow doesn't have to touch your knee.)

6. Exhale.

7. Return to starting position.

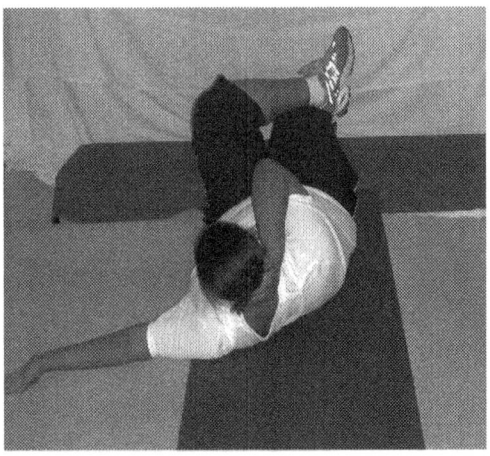

Today's Snack: Ten pretzel sticks with a low-calorie beverage

Day 24: "The Joy of Exercising"

Are you hooked? For the last few weeks, you've moaned and groaned. You've suffered aches and pains. And you've probably been sweaty!

Ah-h-h-h. The joys of exercising.

You have also probably noticed that you are sleeping better, you can stretch farther than before, and you have more energy.

Today's Focus:
Biceps: Four sets of twelve reps. **(Refer to Day 3)**
Triceps: Four sets of twelve reps. **(Refer to Day 3)**
Inner Thigh: **(Refer to Day 21)**
Outer Thigh: **(Refer to Day 21)**

Today's Snack: Five vanilla wafers with 1/2 cup of vanilla pudding

"The Joy of Exercising"

Instead of This Recipe:
Aunt Linnie's Pound Cake

Ingredients
8 eggs
1 lb. butter
2 cups flour
1 box confectionary sugar
2 tbsp. baking powder

Choose This Recipe:
Eight Weeks of Exercising

Ingredients
1 hour of aerobics (bike, jog, walk, or aerobic dance) twice a week
1 hour of strength training
20 minutes of stretching

Preparation Time: Six to eight weeks to see changes

Start with an aerobic activity for thirty minutes twice a week.
Add twenty minutes of strength training twice a week.
By the fourth week, gradually increase aerobics to forty-five minutes and strength training to forty minutes.
Mix in twenty minutes of stretching, yoga, or Pilates.
By the sixth week, add another fifteen minutes of aerobics and strength training.

By choosing the exercise recipe over the pound cake recipe, you will burn 200 calories in one hour instead of eating 200 or more calories in five minutes.

Day 25: Invest in Yourself—Great People Do

<u>Invest in Yourself:</u>
Invest in eating and exercising right.
Invest in getting plenty of sleep.
Invest in meditation or prayer.

<u>Or you can choose to:</u>
Invest in poor eating and exercise habits.
Invest in not getting enough sleep.
Invest in a lack of spiritual wellness, which leads to poor mental and physical health.

Today's Focus: Invest in yourself. Take an aerobics class. Stretch for ten minutes.

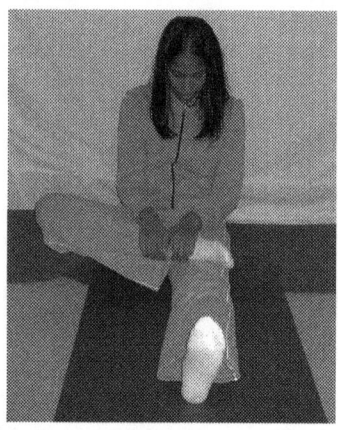

1. Sit down and straighten your legs.
2. Next, cross your right leg over your left leg.
3. Hold position for fifteen to twenty seconds.
4. Breathe naturally.
5. Switch legs.

Today's Snack: Ten baby carrots with 2 tbsp. low-fat cream cheese dip. Blend your favorite fruit or vegetable in the dip.

Short Story Four: Investing in Yourself

Sandra, a thirty-year-old female, came to me in March of 2005 to prepare for the 2005 Honolulu Marathon for AIDS, scheduled for December. At the time, 5' 4" tall Sandra weighed 274 pounds.

I prescribed an exercise program consisting of one hour of strength training twice a week. On her own, Sandra joined the National AIDS Marathon Training Program, where she ran or walked on the weekends. At the end of November 2005, she had lost thirty pounds.

On December 8, 2005, Sandra ran the Honolulu Marathon for AIDS. It took her eight hours. Go, girl!

Today, Sandra is preparing for her second race. She works out in the mornings three times a week at a local gym, she sees me twice a week, and she runs two miles a day on the weekend just to stay in shape.

You don't have to run in a marathon, but investing in yourself is a job that you don't want to waste. It takes time, patience, and consistency to reach your goal. Remember, inch by inch or pound by pound, you will eventually get there.

(Sandra is the model on Day 3)

Day 26: Mind over Matter

You may have heard something similar to the above saying. It is true.

When you finally cannot stand being fat,
When you finally cannot stand being physically out of shape.
When you finally have had enough,
Your mind says, "Enough is enough."
Your mind influences your attitude.
Your attitude changes your behavior.
Your behavior changes you.

Today's Focus:
Biceps: Five sets of twelve reps. (**Refer to Day 3**)
Triceps: Five sets of twelve reps. (**Refer to Day 3**)

Today's Snack: Three graham crackers with 4 oz. of soy milk or 1% milk

How to: Pilates

<u>Position 1</u>
(For those of you using your neck to lift yourself when performing sit-ups). This is a great exercise because it doesn't involve improper lifting of the neck. My clients love this one, and you will get a good workout.

1. Sit down with your legs straight in front of you. Feet are flexed.
2. Place the Fitness Circle between your legs.
3. Place both hands on the handles of the Fitness Circle.
4. Press down three times, and exhale through your mouth with each press.
5. On the fourth press, hold for ten seconds.
6. Release the hold, but keep hands on the Fitness Circle.

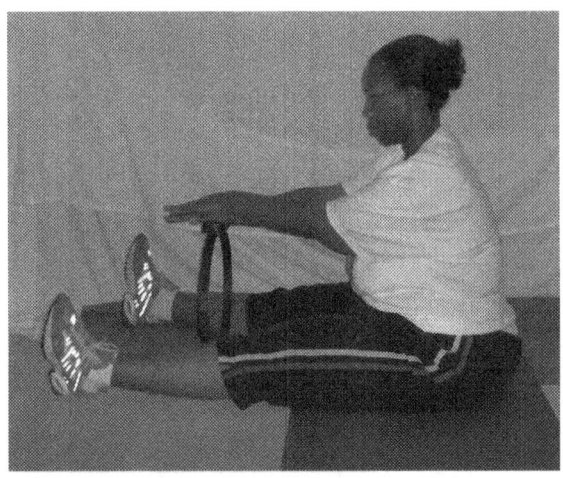

©*This exercise is from STOTT PILATES®, a subsidiary of Merrithew Corporation*

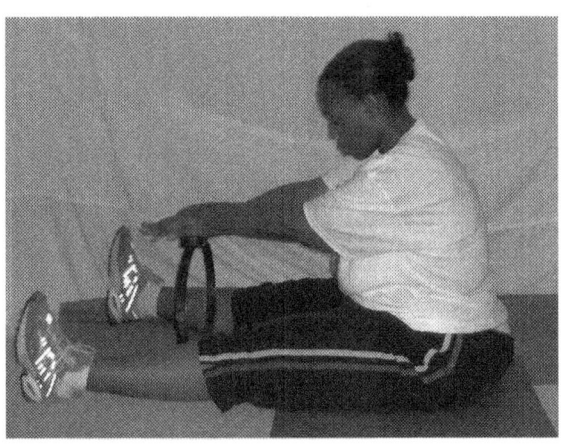

©*STOTT PILATES®, a subsidiary of Merrithew Corporation.*

Position 2

When pressing down keep hands on the Fitness Circle and lean slightly forward.

Day 27: Take Aim

Aim beyond the stars so that if you fall, you will land among the stars, and you will realize how great you have become.

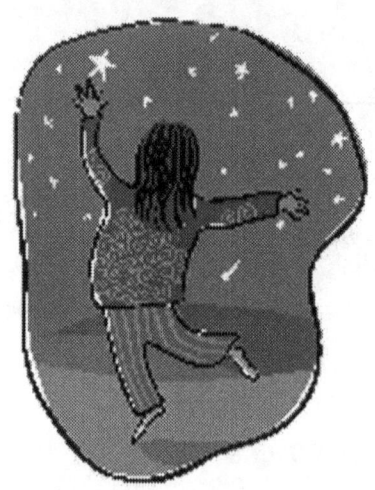

Today's Focus:
Walk for thirty-five minutes. Stretch for ten minutes. (**Refer to Days 5, 6, and 11**)

Target Legs (Inner and Outer Thighs): Four sets of fifteen reps. (**Refer to Day 21**)

Today's Snack: 4-oz. fruit cup and 4 oz. of cottage cheese

Day 28: Absent

Today's Snack: Blend 4 oz. apple juice with a diced banana and 1/2 cup of cantaloupe. A great smoothie!

Day 29: Sh-h-h-h

You are probably wondering why the previous page was blank. Not one thought, phrase or word came to me.

Sometimes there are days when nothing comes into our minds. And we worry that we have become absentminded. But we need those days to throw away the garbage and accomplish other chores on the endless task list we create for ourselves.

We think we always need people around. We can't sleep without the television on.

Perhaps on those quiet days, we can hear God telling us to forget about our lists and let him take over.

Surrender to him.

"I will do the thinking for you," God says.

Sh-h-h-h. Do you hear him? If not, go back and take a long look at the blank page.

"Don't be afraid."

You say you don't get it. What's up with this blank page? Look again.

"I have a box full of your dreams and hopes, yet you don't ask," he says. *"You are too busy looking down, too busy wanting to be the superstar, too busy wanting to do everything yourself. Just too busy. Too busy not including me."*

"You are not alone. You cannot do it all yourself. You see, I am the one who holds the key. If only you take time out to see. I am the superstar. And without me, your dreams will not be fulfilled. So take a break and let me to do the rest."

Today's Focus: Let's stretch.

Today's Snack: A good, hot cup of tea and five sugar-free cookies.

Day 30: Say It Aloud

"I will have one or two enjoyable bites of cheesecake."
Say it aloud.

"I will eat just one slice of pizza."
"I will lose this weight."
"I will exercise today."

Saying it out loud will make you commit to those words.
Words are more powerful when you say them aloud.

Today's Focus:
Bicep Curls: Four sets of twelve reps. (**Refer to Day 3**)
Triceps Kickbacks: Four sets of twelve reps. (**Refer to Day 3**)

Now say it aloud:
"It is my turn to exercise for the next thirty days."

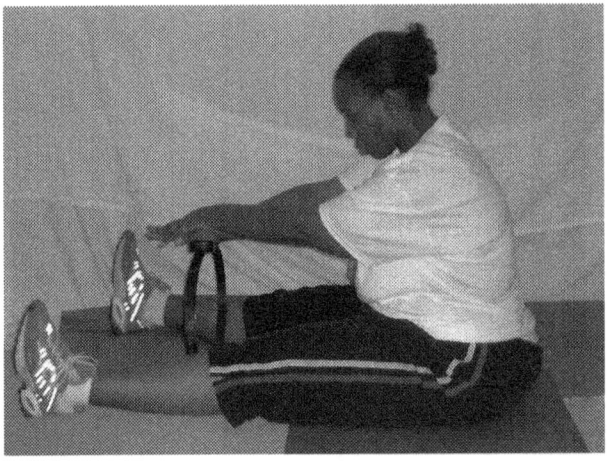

Turn the page.

Day 31: Now It's My Turn

To Plan My Goals:

1._____

2._____

3._____

To Plan My Actions:

1._____

2._____

3._____

To Record My Success:

1._____

2._____

3._____

Today's Snack: _____

Appendices

Helpful Tips

1. Find an exercise you like, and commit to it. Start slowly, and gradually increase your workout.

2. If you walk or run every day, change your shoes every six months to avoid injuries. When your shoes become too comfortable—worn, loosely fitted, with holes or lacking firmness—you need to replace them.

3. Drink water before, during, and after exercise to avoid dehydration. For every pound lost, drink two cups of water.

4. Give yourself plenty of time to warm up and cool down.

5. High impact is not always better. Focus on low-impact exercises to avoid injuries.

6. Exercise during cool times of the day.

7. Wear loose-fitting clothes.

8. Avoid wearing those rubber suits to lose weight. You can become more dehydrated than usual and lose consciousness.

9. If you run outdoors, run with a buddy.

10. Be careful of wearing headphones when exercising outdoors. You need to hear the traffic to avoid accidents and unanticipated surprises.

11. The best time to exercise is any time that is convenient for you. It doesn't matter whether you exercise in the morning, afternoon, or evening; you will burn the same amount of calories. (In hot weather, however, it is best to exercise in the early morning or late afternoon.)

12. Exercise your upper body on Monday, Wednesday, and Friday. For the lower body, exercise on Tuesday, Thursday, and Saturday. Rest on Sunday.

13. Consult with a personal trainer to monitor your technique.

Choices

Do whatever it takes:

- To lose weight
- To tone up
- To strengthen
- To relax

We all have choices.

- Walk or run
- Yoga, Pilates, or stretch class
- Dyna-Band®, weights, or other equipment
- Funk, jazz, or African dance
- Tapes or aerobic classes
- Step or spin
- Swim or water aerobics
- High-impact or low-impact
- Kickboxing or boot camp

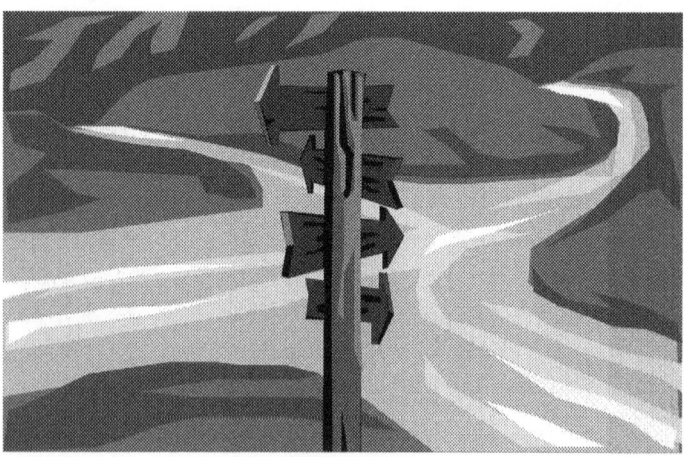

If you don't have equipment:

- Take the stairs.
- Walk around your car or block, or at the local school track.
- Walk, don't shop, at the mall. Walk before the stores open.
- Walk up and down the hallway in your apartment building.
- Go to the grocery store, and walk up and down the aisles.
- Do toe raises at the bus stop.
- Do wall push-ups at home or in your office.

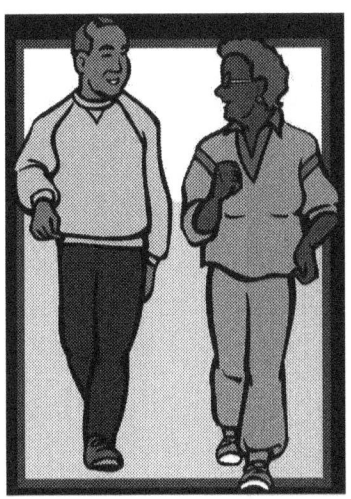

If you don't have weights:

- Use soup cans for bicep curls.
- Do wall or floor push-ups.
- Do squats at the kitchen sink.

- Do lunges over your kitchen broom.
- Push your vacuum a little harder to work your back muscles.
- Take a load of clothes to the laundry room. Lifting the basket several times is a great arm workout.
- Sponsor an exercise party with friends.
- Start a walking program at your place of worship, apartment building, or office.
- Don't forget mental exercises. Meditate at home or at the office. Listen to soft music during your lunch break.

Choices

Every day you make choices. Should you buy your lunch from the fast food place or go to the local health food store? There are consequences to every choice, good or bad. The same applies to choosing foods over the counter, at a restaurant, or at the grocery store. In meal preparation, you make the choice to fry, bake, or broil the food. Bad choices can lead to unwanted pounds.

Food is measured in energy, called calories.

If the number of calories you take in is greater than the amount that you burn, you will be overweight. If the number of calories you take in is less than the number of calories you burn, you will lose weight.

The choice is yours.

Your calories from fat should be 1/3 or less of the total calories.

A calorie from fat is the number of calories from fat in a serving of food.

One 1-oz. bag of pretzels
110 calories
10 calories from fat

One 1-oz. bag of potato chips
150 calories
80 calories from fat

Five salted-top crackers
60 calories
0 calories from fat

Five butter crackers
80 calories
35 calories from fat

1.5-oz. granola bar
90 calories
25 calories from fat

1.5 oz. milk chocolate bar
230 calories
120 calories from fat

The Fork: Proceed with Caution

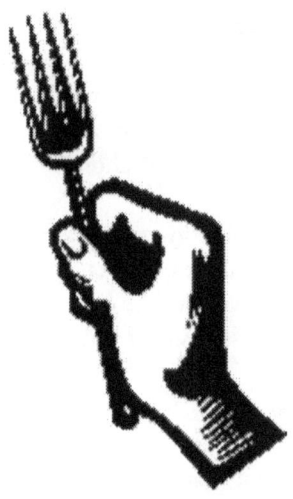

The first forks were large, two-pronged tools (the prongs are called *tines*) that the ancient Greeks used for eating. However, the smaller pieces of food fell through the tines.

During the eleventh century, a Greek princess died after using a fork during her wedding. After this incident, forks were considered scandalous. This is from www.didyouknow.org/forks.

The royal and wealthy families of Spain, Italy, France, and England slowly adapted the design of the fork. During the fourteenth century, France introduced the four-tined fork, which is still in use today. In 1630, Governor Winthrop of Massachusetts introduced the first fork in America.

Today, in the twenty-first century, the fork can be considered a weapon of mass destruction, because it can lead to unwanted pounds. Imagine how many calories, ounces, and pounds of food you shovel to your mouths each day with the fork. Imagine how many more we will consume for the twenty, thirty, forty, or more years left in your lifetime. Wow! That's a lot.

Proceed with caution. Eat smaller portions. With each bite, chew for twenty seconds or longer. Take a deep breath, and wait twenty seconds before the next mouthful.

Proceed with caution. Wait twenty minutes before you decide to eat the second helping.

Proceed with caution. Fill your plate from pots and pans on the stove to avoid temptation at the dinner table. Serving food at the table will make you eat more.

Proceed with caution. If you nibble or taste food at the stove, you must count those calories as part of your daily total. Therefore, eat less at the table.

Proceed with caution. Mothers, don't reach for the food that remains on your child's plate. Those calories count.

Proceed with caution. Cancel your "Clean Your Plate Club" membership.

Portion Control

Food:	The right portion is the size of:
3-oz. meat, fish or poultry	A lady's palm or a bar of soap
1-oz. of cheese	Four dice or one CD case
One slice of bread	Two CD cases
Baked potato	A computer mouse
Apple	A tennis ball
1/4 cup of ice cream	A tennis ball
1 tbsp. of salad dressing	Two thumbs
One cup of broccoli	Your fist
1/2 cup of beans	The first three fingers of your hand

Out of Sight, Out of Mind

I'm sure you, like most of us, have a friend or two who can't understand why she is gaining too much weight, or why she can't seem to lose weight.

Scenario 1:

Let's call her Mollie. She has three children, five to eight years of age. When they arrive home from school at 3:30 PM, Mollie gives them cookies, sodas, and chips in front of the television. She does this because she needs time to get dinner ready for the family.

As she prepares dinner, she tastes to check that the food is properly seasoned. She nibbles on the mashed potatoes, the vegetables, and the meat. She nibbles to make sure her gravy tastes like the gravy her mother makes.

As the dinner cooks, Mollie grabs three chocolate chip cookies from the open bag on the counter without realizing it. She goes into the den to quiet the children. While she's there, she grabs a few chips and drinks four ounces of her oldest daughter's soda.

At 4:45 PM, Mollie calls the family to dinner. She only eats three bites from her own plate but eats leftovers from her youngest daughter's plate.

At 10:00 PM, Mollie stands on the scale and calls out to her husband that the diet the dietitian gave her isn't working.

Can you identify the situations where Mollie has gained extra calories?

1. Tasting food as she cooks.

2. Eating from the cookie bag.

3. Eating her daughter's chips and drinking her soda.

4. Eating food from her youngest daughter's plate.

Scenario 2:

On the way home from work, Sara stops by the local carry-out restaurant, and grabs some dinner. As soon as she arrives home, her best girlfriend calls to ask her out to dinner. Sara accepts the invitation and meets her girlfriend at a restaurant. She orders even though she ate earlier. After all, friends keep friends company.

What is wrong with this story?

Should Sara have stayed home?

No, Sara didn't have to stay home, but she should have ordered a broth soup or a salad with low-fat dressing if she just wanted to keep her friend company.

Avoiding Temptations

- Place those high-calorie snacks on the top shelf and push them to the back, so you will not be able to see them.

- Place snacks and other tempting foods in opaque containers, so you cannot see them.

- If you take snacks to work with you, put them in a snack bag instead of a sandwich bag. (Snack bags are 6 ½" × 3 ¼"; sandwich bags are 6 5/8" × 5 7/8".)

- Serve food from the stove. **When you serve from the table, you eat more**.

- Turn the lights off in the kitchen to remind yourself: **no lights, no food.**

- Brush your teeth right after dinner. This will remind you not to eat.

- When cooking and tasting food, remember, **those calories count, too**!

Eat Less Fat

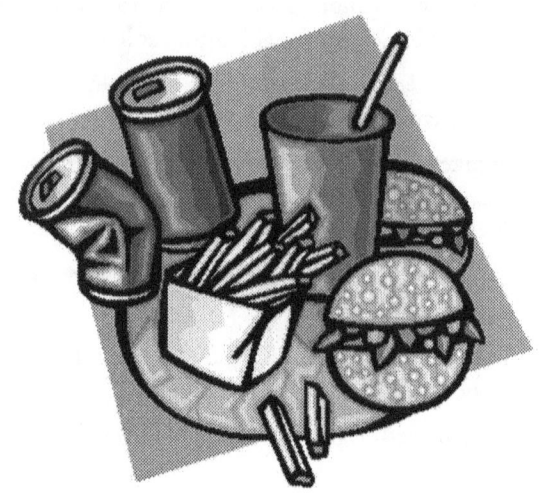

- Use the correct serving size for fat: 1 tsp. margarine or mayonnaise, 1 tbsp. regular salad dressing, gravies, and creams.

- Bake, broil, or poach meats.

- Trim the fat on meats.

- Eat at least six ounces of meat a day. The proper serving size is three ounces, which is about the size of a lady's palm, a deck of cards or a computer mouse.

- Select foods with 0–3 grams of fat per 100 calories.

- Reduce your fat and add more spices to replace the fat taste.

- Your plate should be 3/4 vegetables. About 1/4 of the plate should be protein and fat.

- Use more tomato-based sauces instead of creams.

- Use low-fat or non-fat yogurt to stuff pasta shells.

- Choose low-fat snacks such as fruit or dried fruit.

- Look for 94% fat-free popcorn.
- Choose low-fat pretzels or baked chips as a snack food.
- Look for sugar-free, low-fat cookies.
- Share entrées and ask for sauces/creams on the side.
- Choose part-skimmed ricotta cheese, light cheese, or 50–70% fat-free cheese.
- Eat four to five fruits a day as snacks.
- When baking pizza, add more vegetables and sauce to the bread.
- Add more herbs and spices such as ginger, cilantro, garlic powder (not garlic salt), or celery powder (not celery salt). Add onion to spice up low-fat foods. You can add these spices to fish, chicken, peas, and beans.
- Add Canadian bacon or smoked turkey to season vegetables.
- Mix different greens together to flavor foods. For example, mix collard greens or mustard with kale. Add tomatoes to black-eyed peas. Add diced pineapples and raisins instead of margarine to sweet potatoes.
- Use olive or canola oil instead of butter.
- Limit eggs to no more than three per week.
- Use tub or liquid margarine with no trans-fats (check the label).
- Avoid saturated fats, plastic fats like canned shortening or lard, fatback, and bacon.

Dining Out

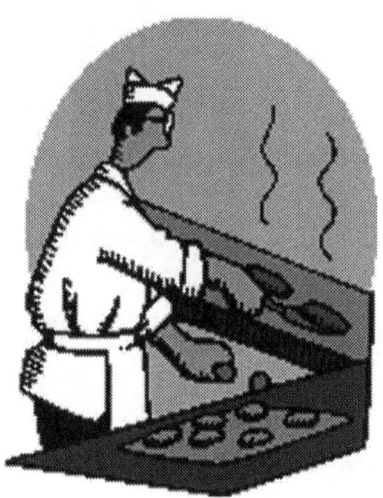

- Plan ahead.
- Call the restaurant to ask whether the menu includes low-fat foods.
- Stick to your meal plan.
- Ask the wait staff for smaller portions. Order any sauces on the side.
- Stick to the "Volumetric Diet": Choose low-calorie soups, low-calorie beverages, salads, and vegetables before selecting your entrée. This will help fill you up on low-calorie, nutrient-dense foods instead of the rich, fatty entrees.
- Order your meats baked, broiled, poached, or stir-fried.
- Pull the skin off the chicken or turkey before eating.
- Pass up the bread, butter, and chips. Order salad instead.
- Choose low-fat salad dressing.

- Bag half of your food first, so you will not be tempted to eat all of it. Save it for another day.
- For dessert, order fruit or sherbet.
- Share high-fat desserts.
- If you order a large sandwich, don't be ashamed to eat only half.
- Order vegetables instead of the baked potato or rice.
- Sipping a low-calorie beverage throughout the night can help you avoid temptation.

Traveling

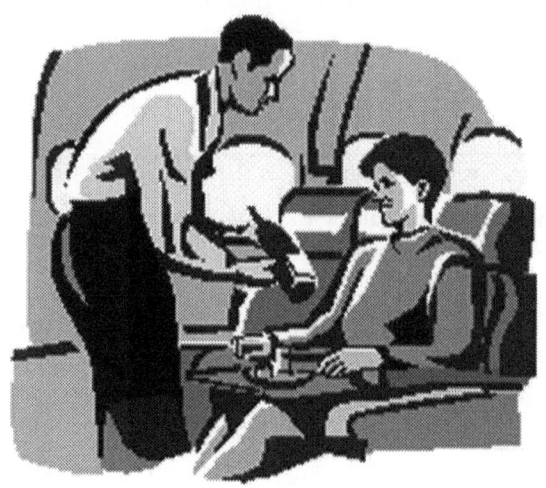

- Plan ahead.
- Take your eating and exercise plans with you.
- At the hotel, visit the gym or walk around the hotel at least ten times.
- When visiting friends, find out whether your gym has a location nearby.
- Take your friends on a walk.
- Carry a healthy snack with you.
- Balance a rich meal with a low-calorie meal.
- On the plane, avoid the salty snacks. They will make you thirsty for a high-calorie drink, and you may not be able to stop at just one.
- When traveling in a car, take a lunch bag or ice chest full of low-calorie, nutrient-dense foods.

- On the train, walk up and down the aisles. Bring your own snacks to avoid the temptation of eating high-fat, high-salt meals.

- Avoid vending machines when traveling. Bring your own fruit or dried fruit.

- Order grilled chicken and a salad with a low-calorie beverage.

- Share the calorie-rich entrées with a friend so you can share the calories.

- When dining out, choose more salads, vegetables, and tomato-based sauces.

- Try not to plan activities around food.

- Eat before you go out.

- Take along an exercise tape and a DVD player to play it.

- Take a Dyna-Band® with you. It can easily be folded into your suitcase or carry-on bag.

- When sightseeing, walk instead of taking a car.

- At buffets, choose the foods without the sauces and heavy creams.

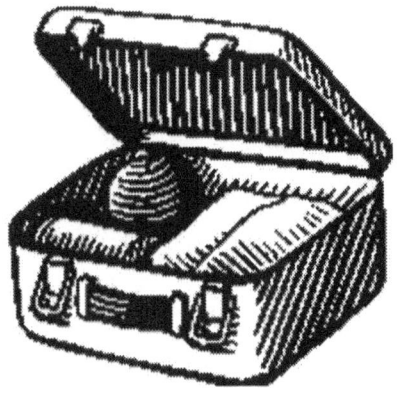

Brown Bag Lunches

Every day, millions of Americans wonder what to fix themselves and their children for lunch. Peanut butter again? One of those high-fat, high-salt frozen entrees, or Oscar Meyer's Lunch Combinations for the kids?

Don't panic. Add pizzazz to your lunches.

- Try chicken or turkey breast with light mayonnaise and sliced seedless grapes on lettuce.

- Try hummus with pita bread or stir-fry vegetables with whole-wheat pita bread.

- Wrap chicken or turkey slices in iceberg lettuce and sprinkle sweet and sour sauce on the wrap.

- Wrap tofu in lettuce and serve with a sauce.

- Add raisins to salad for flavor and texture.

- When making coleslaw, add sliced apples and pineapples to give it a tangy flavor. To lower the fat content, add a low-fat yogurt mix with mayonnaise as dressing.

- Don't be afraid to add extra vegetables to your canned soups.

- For condiments, use mustard, non-fat yogurt, and vinegar. If your children just have to have regular mayonnaise, mixed it with buttermilk or yogurt, and add herbs to spice up the dressing.

- Mix 1/4 cup of peanut butter with 1 tbsp. of honey. Mix well. Cut or dice your favorite fruits and vegetables. Dip your fruits and vegetables into the peanut butter and honey mixture. Bon appétit!

- Brown bag lunches do not have to be boring. Include a special "I love you" note or words of encouragement in lunch bags. Roll up a colorful placemat and include it in the bag. Tell the children and your husband to use it at lunch time. Don't forget yourself. You will be amazed at how simple things make you feel good.

- Making your own lunch saves money and helps you control portion sizes, as well as the amount of fat, sugar, and salt in the meal.

What can you do to make your lunch special?

1._____

2._____

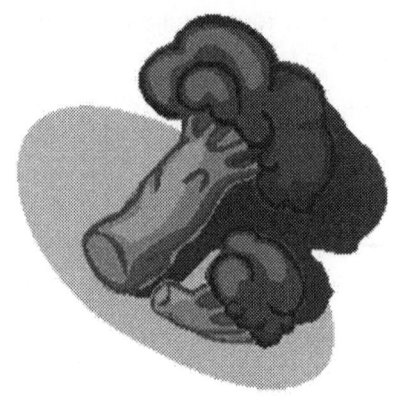

Increase Your Fruits and Vegetables

- Add tomatoes, onions, green peppers, or mushrooms to eggs to make an omelet.

- Add fruits to cereal.

- If you don't drink milk, add fruit cocktail to your cereal. I do. It's good.

- Add warm prune juice to your shredded wheat.

- Add fruit to your muffin or pancake mix.

- Top pancakes with fresh fruit or applesauce.

- Add mixed vegetables to rice or mashed potatoes.

- When cooking rice add cranraisins or mixed vegetables to increase fiber and to add flavor.

- Boil dried apricots in rice water to add flavor.

- Try adding roasted pecans to brown rice for extra crunch, fiber, and flavor.

- Add diced apples or pineapple chucks and yogurt to reduce fat and give a zesty taste to coleslaw.

- Add prunes to your brownie mix to give it a moist texture.
- Add carrots and spinach to your meatloaf.
- Blend zucchini, yellow squash, and acorn squash together. Mix with tomato sauce, and pour over cooked spaghetti. This mixture acts as meat sauce.
- Make mock mashed potatoes with cauliflower. Season to taste.

Don't Salt It, Spice It

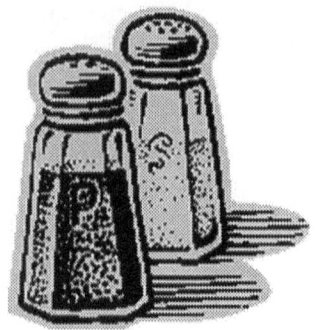 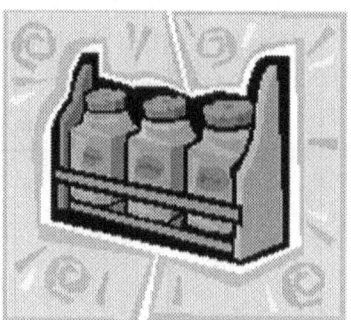

Did you know there are 14,000 uses for salt? Salt is the most common spice used to season foods. It is used in our tap water, processed foods, canned goods, and dried and frozen foods.

Salt is half sodium and half chloride. The recommended daily intake is 2,400 mg, which is equal to one teaspoon.

Studies have shown that a diet high in salt can raise your blood pressure.

So cut back on salt. Use herbs and spices to season your foods.

Basil	Egg, fish, tomato sauce
Bay leaves	Soups, stews, boiled beef and pork
Garlic	Meats, stews, soups, and salads
Oregano	Italian foods and stews
Sage	Poultry, pork, lamb, and stuffing
Beans	Cloves, cumin, mint, onion, green bell pepper
Carrots	Cinnamon, cloves, mint
Lettuce	Basil, dill, lemon
Potatoes	Basil, dill, parsley, bay leaves, rosemary

When adding fresh herbs and spices, use two to three times more than you would with dried herbs. In your soups or stews, add herbs in the last ten minutes of cooking. Cook with herbs when you are cutting back on fat, to replace the flavor.

Use vinegar, pineapple, or orange juice to enhance foods.

Use lemon juice or grate the peel of an orange or lemon to add zest to your dishes. This works particularly well with sweet potatoes.

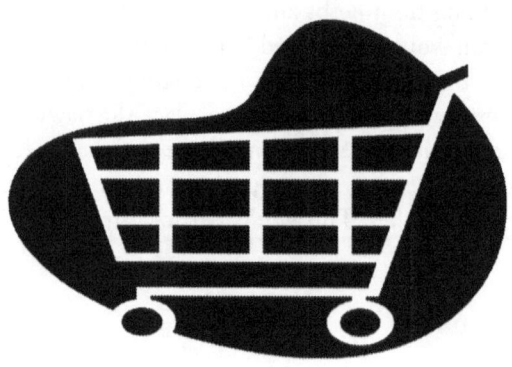

Shopping Tips

- Eat before you go shopping to avoid overspending and buying more than you need.

- Make a list and stick to it.

- Use coupons with store discounts for bigger savings.

- Use coupons for foods you usually buy.

- Let your children pick one or two of their favorite foods.

- Many stores have their own "Savings Card Reward Programs," which offer savings to preferred customers. Obtain a store savings card to take advantage of these savings.

- Buy fresh fruit in season.

- Buy only what you need, especially when you visit the big warehouse stores. The large selection of products at these warehouses may make you spend more.

- Buy fresh vegetables in bulk when they're on sale. Blanch, then cut or dice, and store them in freezer bags for later use. You'll save money and have fresh vegetables whenever you want them.

- Check your local newspaper ads for sales.

- Select lean cuts of meats such as tenderloins, loin chops, or Canadian bacon.

- Limit the amount of duck or goose you eat. These types of poultry are high in saturated fats.

- Buy low-fat or skim dairy products. Buy buttermilk for rich taste low in fat.

- Buy low-fat or part-skim cheese.

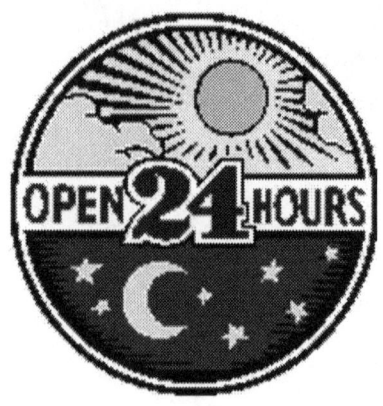

The 24-Hour "Munch-Bug"

You have followed your diet. You have eaten your three meals and a snack. You have just finished working your 3:30 to 11:00 PM shift. It is late, and you are still hungry. *What do you do?*

Everyone has suffered from an attack of the "munchies." You may have tried everything. You've tried calling a friend, drinking plenty of water, even cleaning the house late at night to avoid eating, but the 24-hour "munch bug" has won. You can't stand it any longer.

I don't advocate eating late at night as a rule, but let's be realistic. There are nurses, doctors, firemen, postal workers, police officers, and others who work the night shift.

What do they do?

Eating is necessary in order for the body to function, and I have learned to set realistic goals for my clients who work nights. I advise them to eat low-calorie, nutrient-dense foods to help squash the "munch bug."

Such foods help them resist that leftover pizza, Chinese food, or mom's double-layer chocolate cake.

When you're under attack by the "munch bug," try these low-calorie, nutrient-dense foods:

- 1/2 cup of cereal and a cup of 1% or skim milk
- A slice of low-carb bread with 1/2 tbsp. of peanut butter
- A piece of fruit
- 6 oz. of yogurt
- A small bag of unsalted pretzels with a low-calorie beverage
- Two to three cups of popcorn without butter
- 4 oz. of yogurt with 2 tbsp. of granola
- A shredded wheat biscuit with ten peanuts nuts, toasted for ten minutes
- Half of a banana and 1/2 tbsp. of peanut butter
- 4 oz. of cottage cheese with fruit
- An apple with one slice of part-skim cheese
- 1/2 cup of **gelatin** with 1/2 cup of fruit
- 4-oz. protein smoothie
- 1 oz. of tuna fish with five unsalted crackers
- Frozen popsicles without table sugars

Can you think of anything else?

1._____

2._____

3._____

The New Food Guide Pyramid

It has been thirteen years since the first Food Guide Pyramid was introduced by the USDA (U.S. Department of Agriculture). The new My Pyramid food guidance system is made up of a spectrum of colors, each representing a food group. You will notice that each column differs in size. The larger the column, the more you should eat of that food group. The smallest column, which consists of fats and oils, means that you should eat the least amount of these foods.

My Pyramid's goal is to individualize the MyPyramid plan and make recommendations based on your gender, age, and physical activity levels. The old Food Guide Pyramid represented all sizes and shapes.

One size doesn't fit all. Have a seat at your computer, and go to www.mypyramid.gov or www.usda.gov. Look in the right corner of your screen, and fill in your gender, age, and the number of minutes you exercise every day.

When you have entered your information, the plan will take you to another screen. There, you will read a recommendation based on your entries.

(The site's recommendations are intended as guidelines. For a more accurate assessment, you should see a registered dietitian. The dietitian can develop a personalized meal plan to suit your lifestyle.)

MyPyramid recommends that I consume 2,200 calories daily because I exercise every day. This is an estimate of my needs, based on the new MyPyramid guidelines. My recommended plan includes the following:

Orange (grains)	7 oz. per day
Green (vegetables)	three cups of dark green and orange veggies
Red (fruits)	Two cups (not juice), 15 grapes, half grapefruit, etc.

Blue (milk)   One cup nonfat milk, one slice of
                           cheese, 8 oz. milk, etc.
Purple (meat and beans) 6-oz. (1 tbsp. peanut butter,
                           1/2 oz. nuts, etc.)
Aqua (physical activity)   30 minutes or longer

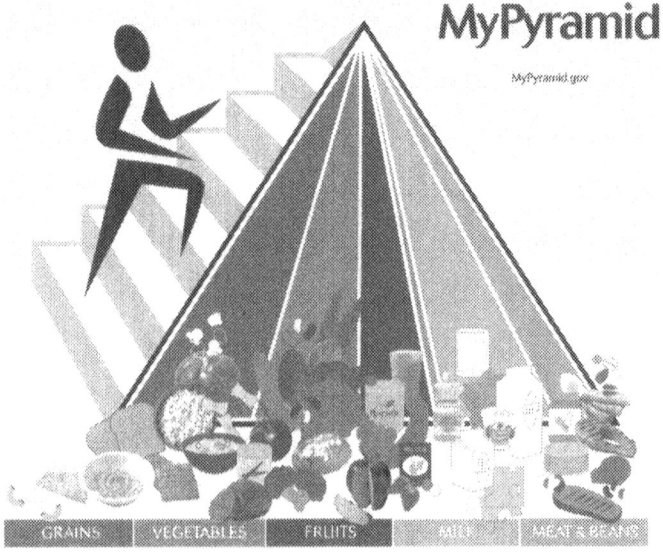

Reprinted with permission from USDA

At www.mypyramid.gov, when you click on a food group, the plan explains about servings and the types of foods you need to eat on a daily and weekly basis.

The new MyPyramid plan provides you with recommendations on your food intake and physical activity, based on information you provide. Visiting the Web site daily can help you make the necessary changes to lose weight and/or eat healthy. MyPyramid is easy to use, and will help jump-start your fitness program.

Now log off, and let's get back to exercising at your chair.

Today's Focus: stretches. (Refer to Days 6, 11, 15, and 17.)

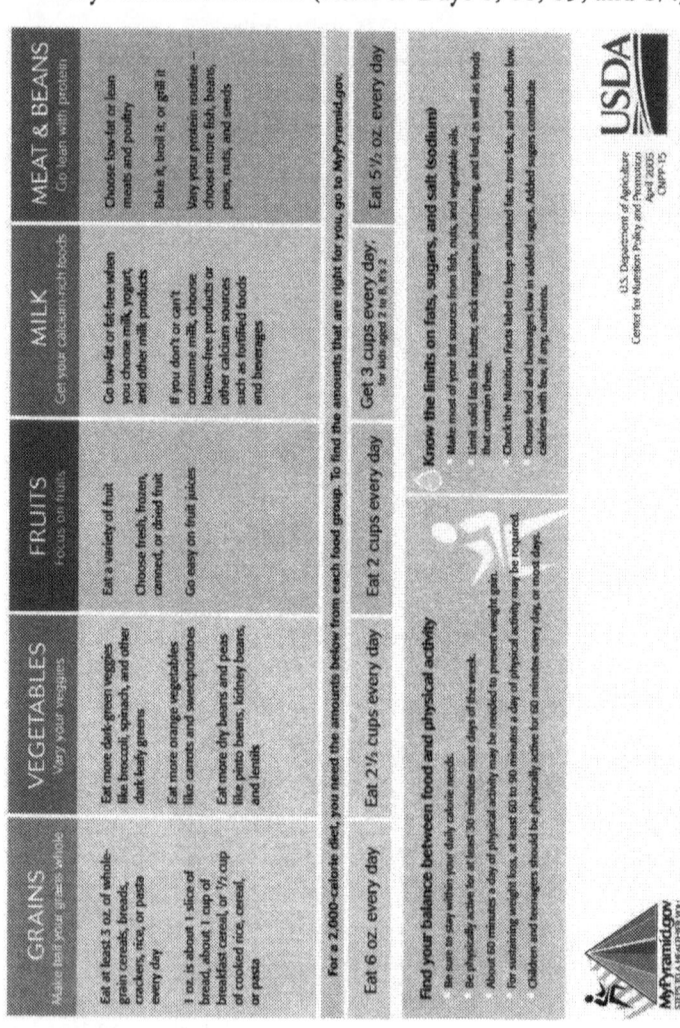

Reprinted with permission from USDA.

Cost Does Matter

I often hear the words, "Healthy foods cost more."
That is true.
Fresh fruits and vegetables cost more for these reasons:

- Food storage costs before they get to the store

- Shipping costs

- Fruits and vegetables are more perishable than meats. If they are bruised during shipping, they spoil faster.

- You must eat lots of fruits and vegetables to feel full, compared to foods high in fat, oils, or sweets.

What would you choose?

Compare:

Two apples	A bag of potato chips
120 calories	130 calories
Cost: $1.00	Cost: $.25 (1-oz. bag)

Most people would buy the chips because of the price. With the chips, you have $.75 left over to buy another food item.

People tend to choose foods based on their pocketbooks, but cheaper foods are usually higher in fats, oils, and sugars. Remember, though, that if you choose to eat a diet high in fats, salt, and sugar, you may eventually face a chronic illness such as obesity, diabetes, hypertension, high blood cholesterol, and some forms of cancer. Have you considered that, sooner or later, you will have to pay the costs associated with such illness?

You will pay in medical bills, doctor's visits, and sick days. In other words, it is better to spend on preventive care than on corrective care.

Although it is difficult to change, you can start slowly by changing one meal at a time. Start with breakfast, and once you have mastered that, move on to lunch and dinner.

Benefits of a healthy diet:

- You will get a variety of minerals, vitamins, and antioxidants.
- A diet high in fiber can reduce your risk of chronic illness.
- A healthy diet will help you lose weight.

A diet high in fat, oils, and sweets:

- Can lead to obesity.
- Obesity can lead to hypertension, heart disease, diabetes, some cancers, joint diseases, and possibly sleep apnea. Taking care of your health is your responsibility, no one else's.

Water

Your body needs water. You can go thirty days without food but just three days without water.

The adult body is composed of sixty percent water. Water helps with digestion and transporting nutrients and oxygen throughout the body. It lubricates joints. Water also maintains the body's normal temperature.

If you are not a plain water drinker, add lemon, lime, or orange slices for flavor.

To prevent dehydration, you must drink six to eight 8-oz. glasses of water every day. If you exercise, it is crucial to drink water before, during, and after your workout.

Drink at least sixteen ounces before exercising, four to eight ounces during your workout, and sixteen ounces after you finish exercising. If you lose one pound after exercise, you must drink two cups of water to replace the lost fluid.

Two cups = Sixteen ounces = One pound

Don't wait to drink water. Signs of dehydration include thirst and yellow urine. Upon rising in the morning, drink two 8-oz. glasses of water. Drink two 8-oz. glasses at all three meals, and you will have consumed 64 ounces of water for the day.

Water is also found in foods, particularly fruits and vegetables. Healthy foods consist of more water. Water has no calories but offers more volume.

For example:

Fifteen grapes
Eating one at a time will make you feel more satisfied.
Grapes are low in calories because they contain a high volume of water.

Fifteen raisins

It takes two to three bites to eat a handful of fifteen raisins. Although you eat them quickly, you are still hungry. And before you know it, you have eaten another fifteen.

Raisins are higher in calories than grapes because they are higher in sugar.

The next time you dine out; choose a salad and a broth soup before eating the main course. The water in both these foods will make you feel full and satisfied, causing you to eat less of the entrée. If you choose a cream soup over a broth soup, a larger portion of your calories will come from fat calories.

Water Content in Foods

Eat more	Water	Eat Less	Water
Grapes	96%	Meats	50–60%
Lettuce	96%	Butter	16%
Celery	95%	Almonds	4%
Carrots	87%	Oil	No water
Oranges	26%		
Apples	16%		

Choose foods higher in water because they contain fewer calories.

Holiday Eating

'Twas the night before Christmas, and all through the house…visions of sugar plums, grandma's candied yams, Uncle Ed's mashed potatoes loaded with butter, and Aunt Emma's pound cake made with nine eggs danced in my head.

All those holiday goodies do not have to add extra pounds.

You can eat well and still enjoy your holiday favorites, even those rich desserts. The key is to balance high-fat choices with low-fat choices, such as angel food cake with strawberries on top instead of Aunt Emma's pound cake.

Make mashed potatoes with low-fat, low-sodium chicken broth instead of milk, or use mashed cauliflower.

Try using low-fat sour cream mixed with low-fat yogurt for your cream dips.

Blend red kidney beans with cumin and jalapeño peppers to make a dip.

Serve roasted shredded wheat squares sprinkled with grated parmesan cheese for a great low-fat, high-fiber snack. Bake pita bread and serve with hummus.

Add mashed bananas to your favorite candied yams instead of loading the yams with sugar.

Serve low-calorie beverages.

And, if you are traveling from one relative's house to another, eat small meals. For instance, at Aunt Emma's, help yourself to her yams with vegetables. At Uncle Ed's house, have the meat and vegetables. This will help you pace yourself, and you won't hurt anyone's feelings.

Happy Holidays!

About the Author

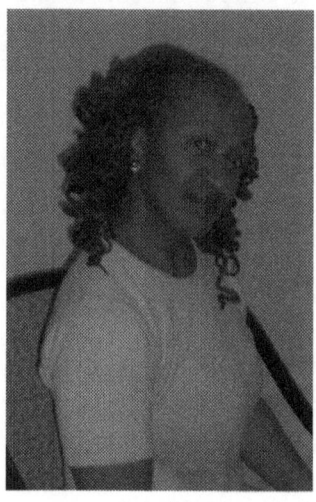

Renee Wiggins, fitness professional and lecturer, is a Certified Personal Trainer, Licensed Certified Massage Therapist, Licensed Dietitian, and owner of Results By Renee, a wellness company located in Silver Spring, Maryland. Ms. Wiggins promotes the advantages of a healthy lifestyle and specializes in designing Personal Lifestyle Programs that motivate, teach, and coach people on how to achieve their optimum health potential.

You can reach Ms. Wiggins through her Web site, by e-mail, or by phone.

E-mail: renee@resultsbyrenee.com
Phone: 301-434-5461
Web site: www.resultsbyrenee.com

Footnotes

Thanks for giving me permission:

©STOTT PILATES ®, a subsidiary of Merrithew Corporation (Day 26)

MyPyramid.gov USDA Center for Nutrition Policy and Promotion (pgs. 86–89)

ClipArt from ©MicroSoft

Fitness Wholesale for use of the Dyna-Band® in the picture.

Resources

Jodi Stolove

Chair Dancing® International Inc.
www.chairdancing.com

Videos
"CHAIR YOGA",
"SIT DOWN & TONE UP"—

978-0-595-38647-5
0-595-38647-4